Overcoming Self-Harm and Suicidal Thoughts

A Practical Guide for the Adolescent Years

In memory of all those who could no longer see the light of hope.

Overcoming Self-Harm and Suicidal Thoughts

A Practical Guide for the Adolescent Years

Liz Quish

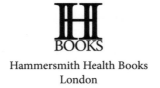

Hammersmith Health Books
London

First published in 2015 by Hammersmith Health Books – an imprint of
Hammersmith Books Limited
14 Greville Street, London EC1N 8SB, UK
www.hammersmithbooks.co.uk

British Library Cataloguing in Publication Data: A CIP record of this book
is available from the British Library.

Print ISBN 978-1-78161-056-5
Ebook ISBN 978-1-78161-057-2

Commissioning editor: Georgina Bentliff
Designed and typeset by: Julie Bennett, Bespoke Publishing Ltd
Cover design by: Julie Bennett, Bespoke Publishing Ltd
Index: Dr Laurence Errington
Production: Helen Whitehorn, Path Projects Ltd
Printed and bound by: TJ International Ltd, UK

Contents

Acknowledgements   vi
Introduction   vii

Chapter 1   Understanding 'self-defeatist syndrome'   1

Chapter 2   Self-harm   13

Chapter 3   Suicide   31

Chapter 4   Talk therapies   49

Chapter 5   Complementary therapies   75

Chapter 6   Eating well for mental health   91

Chapter 7   Parenting   105

Chapter 8   Bereavement through suicide   119

Appendix   133
References and Bibliography   145
Index   151
About the Author   160

Acknowledgements

I would like to extend my gratitude to Mary Mulcahy and Catherine Anne O'Connell, two exceptional and passionate facilitators on the Adlerian Psychology Programme at LIT Tipperary. Thank you both for your encouragement and validation and sparking what has now become my passion.

I would also like to thank the teaching staff of PCI College for their support and feedback as I worked tirelessly to achieve my Counselling and Psychotherapy Degree. A special note of thanks to one of my core lecturers, Willie Egan; your sense of humour and compassion are admirable. Thank you for displaying such empathy, congruence and unconditional positive regard!

Dr Fergus Heffernan, you are a true inspiration and a very special person; thank you for sharing your life story and insights. I learned so much from you and will be eternally grateful that our paths crossed.

My practice supervisors, Marie O'Connor and Frances Burke, thank you for listening, encouraging, validating and gently challenging me.

To my parents and siblings Sean, Mary and Steven, thank you for all that you taught me long before I learned the theory!

To Paul, my husband, thank you for believing in me, for all the cups of tea, and for feeding me as I endeavoured to complete this book. Thank you for making me realise that dreams can and do come true.

Sincere gratitude to Georgina of Hammersmith Books for realising the importance of the subject matter of this book.

Introduction

During my training in Counselling and Psychotherapy I became very interested in self-harming and suicide due to its prevalence worldwide and as such conducted a great deal of research into the topic and engaged in further training in the area. Immediately after I qualified as a Counsellor and Psychotherapist I secured a position as a counsellor with a Self-Harm and Suicide Intervention Crisis Centre based in Ireland.

Through supporting stressed and distressed teenagers from 12 years upwards, I noticed common themes, presentations, thought processes and struggles which I have come to term 'self-defeatist syndrome'. Many came to see me feeling anxious, scared, tired, overwhelmed, angry and isolated, with a very negative view of themselves and their abilities and a great sense of hopelessness and inadequacy. They could not see the beauty within them; it was clouded and forgotten, shadowed by thoughts of uselessness and feelings of inadequacy. There was no brightness or twinkle in their young eyes. Self-defeatist syndrome had taken hold and what I call 'the Gremlin' had moved in and taken over their young minds and souls, causing havoc in their lives. These young teenagers did not know how to evict the Gremlin; many didn't even know it had moved in. You see, the Gremlin is stress that progresses to distress – not a mental illness, but psychological distress that manifests in what I term self-defeatist syndrome.

This syndrome – or collection of symptoms and features that tend to occur together – causes our teenagers to become anxious, angry, hopeless, depressed, and to engage in self-harming; many consider and, unfortunately for some, complete suicide. In my experience, by employing an integrative approach which addresses the teenager's lifestyle, with a focus on nutrition, complementary therapies, talk therapy, exercise and community engagement, self-defeatist syndrome can be defeated and the Gremlin evicted!

I aim to guide readers through the steps and tasks of assisting a teenager in managing and overcoming the many challenges presented by this syndrome, with the ultimate goal of restoring mental wellbeing and family cohesion.

Sadly, self-defeatist syndrome has proven fatal and resulted in many young people worldwide completing suicide, with devastating consequences for their families and friends. In the final chapter of this book I address the impact of such a loss and guide readers through how to support those bereaved by the death of a loved one through suicide.

Chapter 1

Understanding 'Self-Defeatist Syndrome'

A person whose head is bowed and whose eyes are heavy cannot look at the light.

Christine de Pizan

What I will term 'self-defeatist syndrome' throughout this book is the uninvited Gremlin that moves into young minds, metaphorically speaking. The Gremlin is STRESS that leads to DISTRESS, an unruly tenant that is powerful, deceitful and controlling. Its ultimate goal is to take control of a teenager's life in a destructive manner causing him/her to feel alone, depressed, angry, afraid, hopeless and anxious. The Gremlin is not a friend; the sooner it is evicted the better. The longer it stays the more powerful it becomes, taking the teenager hostage. The Gremlin's goal is to isolate the teenager from family and friends, thus making itself even more powerful. It wants to make the teenager feel lonely and powerless, surrendering to the darkness, diminishing his/her light and self-esteem, distorting his/her belief system and sense of self.

The sense of self

The 'self' relates to our uniqueness and individuality, our thoughts, feelings, perceptions and sense of worth, and how we view ourselves. The self also relates to our sense of identity, our

1

belief system and values.

A teenager with a healthy sense of self will:

- ✓ feel confident and competent
- ✓ feel a sense of belonging and acceptance
- ✓ feel secure, safe and valued
- ✓ have self-discipline and self-control
- ✓ learn from and move on from mistakes with new awareness
- ✓ value his/her strengths and accept his/her weaknesses
- ✓ have a healthy set of core values.

These are all the traits that the Gremlin of self-defeatist syndrome despises and wants to eliminate. The Gremlin does not want the teenager to have a healthy sense of self; a healthy sense of self is its enemy. Its wish and desire is for the teenager to have a defeatist view of him/herself. In achieving this, the Gremlin has accomplished its objective and is actively compromising the wellbeing of teenagers, who are not strong enough to evict the Gremlin on their own.

The defeatist attitude

The 'defeatist attitude' refers to an attitude or view of oneself which is negative, pessimistic and unforgiving. A teenager with a defeatist view of him/herself will present with low self-esteem and a noticeable and ongoing lack of motivation, generally deriving little pleasure from life, with a distinct lack of belief in his/her abilities. This is a clear sign that the Gremlin has moved in and taken the teenager hostage. Teenagers in this situation will often use phrases like:

- ✓ What's the point?
- ✓ It won't work for me.

✓ They would all be better off without me.
✓ It's just one thing after another.
✓ I couldn't be bothered.
✓ I can't manage this anymore.
✓ I am no good.
✓ No one cares about me.
✓ I can't do it.

Syndrome

A 'syndrome' refers to a combination of signs and symptoms that are indicative of a particular condition. A teenager in the midst of self-defeatist syndrome will generally present with:

✓ Low energy
✓ Low self-esteem
✓ Depression
✓ Anxiety
✓ Anger
✓ Self-harming
✓ Suicidal ideation (thinking).

Low energy

A teenager can experience low energy for a number of reasons. Adolescence is a period marked by a rapid increase in physical and emotional development. Puberty, hormonal changes and the soaring growth of bones and muscles can have a temporary effect on energy levels, causing many teenagers to feel fatigued from time to time; this is totally normal and to be expected. However, if low energy persists and negatively affects the quality of life of a teenager, a detailed and comprehensive medical investigation is warranted and strongly advised. A full medical investigation should uncover any organic reasons for fatigue and low energy;

then, the right treatment can get a teenager's energy levels back on track and prevent the onset of self-defeatist syndrome.

Common organic reasons for low energy uncovered through a medical investigation in teenagers include:

✓ Infection
✓ Virus
✓ Iron-deficiency anaemia
✓ Low thyroid function
✓ Vitamin B and C deficiencies
✓ Allergies.

Harder to diagnose, and more unusual in younger people, are underactive thyroid (hypothyroidism) and pernicious anaemia/ vitamin B12 deficiency.

If after a full medical investigation no organic causes for low energy and fatigue can be detected, then lifestyle needs to be further scrutinised and addressed as the Gremlin may be actively trying to move in.

Exploring a teenager's lifestyle

Diet

Nutrition is especially important during the adolescent years due to the rapid growth and progression that occurs during this developmental period. Many teenagers have developed poor eating habits and have little understanding of healthy eating and the effect food has on their physical and mental health.

Food production and manufacturing techniques have changed considerably in the last few decades. This, combined with fast-paced lifestyles and an ever increasing reliance on processed foods, has resulted in the decline of fresh and nutritious foods in our diet, particularly in teenagers. Teenagers who have poor eating habits, or who are eating irregularly and consuming lots of processed, high-sugar foods and drinks, are compromising their wellbeing. These foods have a remarkably negative effect on energy levels. Sugary foods and drinks cause energy rushes, but we need to remember that what goes up must come down! These processed and high-sugar foods and drinks give a short bust of energy, but then comes the low. In cases where diet is inadequate and affecting the overall wellbeing of a teenager, parents are advised to consult a nutritionist in order to assess and address their child's negative eating habits. Diet will be addressed in more detail in Chapter 6 (see page 91).

Sleep

When sleep requirements are not being met on an ongoing basis, teenagers will present with fatigue, low energy, exhaustion and a lack of motivation. It is generally recommended that teenagers get eight to 10 hours quality sleep a night. This is vital for the body to relax, repair and refuel. Lack of sleep has a domino effect and impedes mental and physical wellbeing, inviting the onset of self-defeatist syndrome. As I have said already, parents are advised to take their child to a GP to rule out any organic causes of fatigue. In instances where no organic cause is established it is highly likely that the Gremlin has moved in. The Gremlin loves and thrives on the darkness. It becomes alert and active, coming out to play its evil games at night when we are programmed to relax, unwind and fall into a peaceful slumber. The Gremlin is very powerful and demanding, wanting to keep us awake, bolstering and encouraging negative thinking, which leads to rumination, tossing and turning and feeling like our head is going to explode! Thoughts are negative, racing and exhausting. It is vital that teenagers who have been taken hostage by the Gremlin receive appropriate support and professional intervention so they may be facilitated in developing the tools and techniques needed to evict the Gremlin. This will be outlined in Chapter 4 on Talk therapies (see page 49).

Low self-esteem

Self-esteem relates to how we think and feel about ourselves. Teenagers with low self-esteem will not like any part of themselves. This is not the same as not liking an aspect of ourselves, which we can all relate to and generally accept. They will be very critical of themselves and will not be able to identify any positive traits; in this instance, the Gremlin is winning and achieving its objective.

The main characteristics of low self-esteem are:

- ✓ Withdrawal
- ✓ Insecurity
- ✓ Poor body image
- ✓ Isolation
- ✓ Lack of motivation
- ✓ Anger
- ✓ Inability to accept a compliment
- ✓ Self-neglect
- ✓ No value put on own opinion
- ✓ Negative thinking
- ✓ Extremely critical of self
- ✓ Self-blame.

I have witnessed on a daily basis the pain and anguish caused by low self-esteem and how it cripples the emotional and social wellbeing of teenagers.

Reasons for low self-esteem include:

- ✓ Struggling with sexual identity
- ✓ Pressure from parents to achieve, and being likened unfavourably to a sibling
- ✓ Pressure from teachers to achieve high grades
- ✓ Isolation by peer group

✓   Sexual abuse
✓   Physical abuse
✓   Emotional abuse
✓   Being overweight
✓   Being underweight
✓   Break-up of a relationship
✓   Bullying
✓   Rejection.

The Gremlin is very happy and content when it discovers a teenager has experienced, and is struggling with, any of these issues. It taps into this vulnerability with great energy and enthusiasm and feeds the negativity and sense of hopelessness that can emerge from such struggles, further exacerbating the issue. Low self-esteem is the foundation stone of self-defeatist syndrome and results in teenagers becoming depressed, anxious, and angry, engaging in self-harm and contemplating suicide.

Depression

Teenagers who feel depressed will have ongoing low mood, low energy and difficulty concentrating, and often have bouts of sleep disturbances along with tearful and angry outbursts. They will have a poor sense of self, presenting to health professionals with low self-esteem and actively engaging in negative thinking, stating and believing that they are no good, unloved and a burden, and are full of self-loathing. They may lose pride in their appearance and eating or, indeed, begin to overeat for comfort. A teenager experiencing a period of depression will find little pleasure in life and may have ongoing suicidal thoughts and actively engage in self-harming.

A diagnosis of depression is usually made if the symptoms outlined have been persistently present for two to four weeks, or longer. In this instance, self-defeatist syndrome has taken hold and professional intervention is vital. Teenagers who are feeling depressed need support, guidance and patience. They are not able to simply 'snap out' of this state of mind and evict the Gremlin; if they could, believe me they would! The anguish caused by depression is soul destroying. Cognitive behavioural therapy (discussed in Chapter 4 on Talk therapies (see page 49)) is often the talk therapy of choice in supporting a teenager through depression. This form of therapy has been scientifically proven to be extremely beneficial in supporting teenagers through the management of depression. Medication has its place, and parents are advised to seek guidance from their GP around this. It is, however, worth noting that anti-depression medications have many side-effects and can increase and heighten the symptoms for which the medication has been prescribed to treat. Lifestyle habits and choices also need to be addressed in order to manage rather than exacerbate the condition.

Anxiety

Teenagers who present with anxiety are in a constant state of high alert and fearfulness. They are physically and mentally drained as a result of being in this constant state of 'fight or flight'. They experience and struggle with poor concentration, lack of recall, and restlessness, often reporting tension headaches and stomach cramps. Anxiety is a major characteristic of self-defeatist syndrome.

We all have experienced anxiety from time to time, be it before an exam or job interview, moving house, or moving to a new school or job. We feel butterflies in our stomach and may have one or two nights of restless sleep. This type of anxiety is short lived, common and expected in these situations. By contrast, the anxiety that is associated with self-defeatist syndrome is much more debilitating and often and goes hand in hand with depression. Anxiety and depression are best friends that fight

8

us in order to stay together, as together they are more powerful in controlling us. This form of anxiety is constant, draining and debilitating. The body and mind are in a constant state of stress.

Characteristics of chronic anxiety are:

- ✓ Tension headaches
- ✓ Stomach cramps
- ✓ Chest pain
- ✓ Feelings of impending loss of control
- ✓ Tearfulness
- ✓ Physical and mental tiredness and restlessness
- ✓ Nightmares
- ✓ Low levels of concentration
- ✓ Angry outbursts
- ✓ Sweating and feeling clammy
- ✓ Panic attacks.

The wellbeing of a teenager who displays this level of anxiety is highly compromised and entering a danger zone. Many in this situation are also engaging in self-harm and have strong suicidal ideation. They are in a very distressed state, afraid, tired and vulnerable, and in many cases misunderstood by family, friends and teachers.

Many teenagers try very hard to hide their anxiety. They display what I term 'swan stance', appearing to be controlled, confident and at peace on the outside, but underneath they are paddling like crazy, possibly engaging in self-harm in order to release their inner turmoil, if only momentarily. Self-harm will be explored in more detail in Chapter 2 (see page 13).

Anger

Anger is generally a result of an unmet need, perceived or real. The key to managing the anger strand of self-defeatist syndrome is to help teenagers to uncover and verbalise their unmet need in a proactive, healthy, respectful way rather than in an aggressive, reactive manner such as bullying, destructiveness, threats, unpredictability and vengeance.

Teenagers who display regular bouts of anger often, in my experience, have a limited emotional vocabulary; consequently they are unable to identity their feelings and as a result act out, flipping the lid or losing the head. When we are angry and act on this feeling we are in essence switching off the cognitive, logical part of our brain and exposing the more primitive, emotional part and setting it in motion. I am sure we can all recall a situation in which we got angry, acted out and regretted it later! We flipped the lid, exposed our primitive emotional brain and operated without logic – never a good idea!

Pre-menstrual tension may also be a cause of irritability and angry outbursts in girls and women and must be given due consideration. Starflower oil has shown favourable results in counteracting the effects of PMT. It contains gamma linoleic acid, a fatty acid that aids the regulation of hormonal imbalances, thereby reducing tension and anxiety. Parents are advised to seek advice from their GP before deciding to give their child any supplement, particularly if they are taking prescribed medications or other supplements.

Self-harm

Self-harm is the intentional act of harming oneself in order to release inner turmoil and is a very secretive act. It is a flawed coping mechanism in which teenagers engage to release inner anguish and distress as they are unable, or afraid, to express verbally how they are feeling. Engaging in self-harm can cause more distress as the person embarks on a vicious cycle of trying to hide his/her wounds and scars coupled with feelings of guilt and shame, thus exacerbating the distress and turmoil that prompted the self-harming initially.

Acts of self-harm include:

✓   Cutting
✓   Scratching
✓   Breaking bones
✓   Biting
✓   Pulling out hair
✓   Hitting self
✓   Burning self
✓   Poisoning.

The teenager who is engaging in any of these self-harming activities is very distressed, and as such self-defeatist syndrome is extremely active. Self-harm will be explored in more detail in Chapter 2 (see page 13).

Suicidal thinking ('ideation')

'Suicidal ideation' is the term used to describe thoughts about ending a person's own life. These can range from fleeting thoughts to active planning.

A teenager who has suicidal ideation is extremely vulnerable and distressed and in need of immediate attention. Suicidal ideation warrants immediate professional intervention as this means self-defeatist syndrome is highly active and can be fatal. When the light of hope starts to go out, sadly suicide can appear very inviting. Suicide will be explored in more detail in Chapter 3 (see page 31).

Factors associated with the onset of self-defeatist syndrome

There can be many reasons for the onset of self-defeatist

syndrome. It is usually more likely to manifest in teenagers who are greatly distressed due to:

- ✓ Sexual abuse
- ✓ Physical abuse
- ✓ Emotional abuse
- ✓ Bereavement
- ✓ Parental illness
- ✓ Parental addiction
- ✓ Peer bullying
- ✓ Peer isolation
- ✓ Exam pressure and failure
- ✓ Sexual identity confusion
- ✓ Parental separation or divorce
- ✓ Authoritarian parenting
- ✓ 'Parentification', in which the teenager takes on the parenting role for younger siblings
- ✓ Pre-menstrual tension.

Self-defeatist syndrome has many causes and characterises, and can take time to overcome and deal with. It can be very powerful and demobilising. However, the good news is that this syndrome does not have to be fatal; it can be managed and defeated. With early detection and the right blend of interventions the Gremlin can be evicted and peace of mind and inner harmony can be restored.

Chapter 2

Self-harm
– the painful and misunderstood consequences of 'self-defeatist syndrome'

Unexpressed emotions will never die. They are buried alive and will come forth later in uglier ways.

Sigmund Freud

This chapter will provide you with a detailed overview of self-harming in the hope that it will enable you to better understand why it happens and how to manage it most effectively, whether you are a parent or a professional working with teenagers.

Understanding self-harm

A teenager who engages in the act of self-harm is communicating a high level of distress and vulnerability.

Self-harm is often referred to as:

- ✓ Self-injury
- ✓ Self-mutilation
- ✓ Para-suicide
- ✓ Self-abuse
- ✓ Self-inflicted injury.

Self-harm is best described as the deliberate and intentional act of inflicting injury on oneself for the purpose of releasing inner emotional distress, more often than not with no suicidal intent.

The World Health Organisation (WHO) defines self-harm as:

'An act with non-fatal outcome in which an individual deliberately initiates a non-habitual behaviour, that without intervention from others will cause self-harm, or deliberately ingests a substance in excess of the prescribed or generally recognised therapeutic dosage, and which is aimed at realising changes that the person desires via the actual or expected physical consequences.'

Reasons behind the act of self-harming

Reasons behind the act of self-harming include:

- ✓ Struggling with sexual identity
- ✓ Low self-esteem
- ✓ Bereavement
- ✓ Isolation
- ✓ Sexual abuse
- ✓ Physical abuse
- ✓ Emotional abuse
- ✓ Ending of a relationship
- ✓ Transitions (for example, new school)
- ✓ Parental separation and divorce
- ✓ Exam pressure
- ✓ Bullying
- ✓ Rejection by peers
- ✓ Depression
- ✓ Anxiety
- ✓ Addiction
- ✓ Psychological disorder.

It can be extremely challenging for some of us to understand why a teenager would deliberately harm him/herself. You may wonder how physically hurting yourself could make you feel better; if anything, would it not make you feel worse? In my work supporting teenagers who self-harm, the following reasons for this behaviour have emerged:

✓ Inducing a sense of release
✓ Validating inner pain
✓ Giving a sense of control over a situation they feel they have no control over
✓ Helping them to stay alive by giving a momentary release from the distress that might otherwise lead them to consider or complete suicide.

As I have said, self-harm is a means of communicating and releasing distress and inner turmoil. Teenagers engage in this act as a way of coping, not necessarily as a means or desire to end their lives. Many teenagers in this level of distress do not want to die but simply want the emotional pain to end and the act of self-harming gives them a momentary release.

Acts of self-harm

Acts of self-harm include the following:

✓ Cutting
✓ Scratching
✓ Picking skin
✓ Biting
✓ Burning
✓ Pulling out hair
✓ Hitting
✓ Punching

✓ Pinching
✓ Head banging
✓ Over-rubbing of the skin
✓ Body bashing
✓ Poisoning
✓ Interfering with wound healing.

Cutting

In supporting teenagers who engage in self-harming, I have found that cutting is one of the most common forms used by this age group. The most common places for cutting are the wrists, inner arm, inner thighs and stomach. Teenagers tend to cut themselves in places that they can hide. The biggest concern with cutting is that a teenager may unintentionally sever a main artery, which can be fatal. Cutting can also lead to serious infection if wounds are not treated in a timely and appropriate manner.

Objects used to cut include:

✓ Blades
✓ Knives
✓ Scissors
✓ Broken CDs
✓ Broken glass
✓ Paper clips
✓ Staples
✓ Compass
✓ Flattened cans
✓ Sharp pencils
✓ Hair accessories
✓ Pins.

Generally, any object that presents a sharp edge that can scrape or penetrate skin may be utilised.

Scratching

We generally scratch because we have an itch; we scratch and the itch subsides. In the case of self-harm, teenagers will scratch even though they do not have an itch and often break their skin due to the force and repetition used to alleviate their distress.

Picking skin

'Excoriation disorder' is the repetitive and compulsive picking of skin, which results in tissue damage. The region most commonly picked is the face; in this case you have a very clear indicator. Other locations include arms, legs, back, gums, lips, shoulders, scalp, stomach, chest, fingernails, cuticles and toenails.

Biting

Teenagers who bite themselves generally do so in areas that can be easily hidden, usually the inside of the forearm. In some instances, the teenager may intentionally break the skin, which can lead to infection. In my experience, teenagers generally bite themselves when they are very frustrated and annoyed with themselves.

Burning

Burning is a form of self-harm that can be easily passed off as an accident, so you need to be diligent if you notice these 'accidents' are recurring. This may be active self-harm.

Pulling out hair

'Trichotillomania' is the act of intentionally pulling out clumps of hair, be it on the head, eyelashes or eyebrows. Some teenagers pull out their pubic hair, which obviously is easier to hide and may in some instances be an indication of sexual abuse. Hair pulling appears in my experience to be more prevalent in girls than boys. Girls can hide this act more easily through using hair extensions and hair accessories, false eyelashes and pencilling in eyebrows.

Hair loss can sometimes be confused with alopecia. Alopecia is due to a systemic autoimmune disorder in which the body attacks its own hair follicles and suppresses or stops hair growth.

Hitting

Teenagers who hit themselves do so with the intention of altering a current negative state. Many of the teenagers I have worked with reported hitting themselves on the face and head when feeling angry, overwhelmed and frustrated.

Punching

Teenagers who punch themselves generally punch their head, face and stomach.

Pinching

Teenagers may pinch themselves on any part of their body but most commonly will target the face, hands, arms, thighs and stomach. Pinching is done with great force and causes the skin to become very red; it can result in bruising or breaking of the skin.

Head banging

Teenagers who engage in head banging often report ongoing headaches, stiffness in their necks and dizziness. They commonly bang their heads on walls or may rock forwards and backwards, focusing on the exaggerated movement of their head back and forth.

Poisoning

Self-poisoning or overdosing is the act of deliberately consuming a substance in excess of the prescribed dosage. It includes the ingestion or injection of illegal drugs and ingesting or inserting, in some cases through the anus, a non-digestible substance or object. In my experience, over-dosing is much more common in females than males.

Teenagers who are prescribed anti-depressant medications need to be monitored and supervised. Having easy access to these medications can increase the chance of overdosing when feeling low and vulnerable. Overdosing can prove fatal. Other acts of self-poisoning include drinking bleach and inhaling tins of deodorants by spraying in a confined unventilated space.

Over-rubbing of skin

'Over-rubbing the skin' describes the act of excessively rubbing the skin until burn-like friction marks appear. It is generally noted on the hands, lower arms and thighs.

Body bashing

'Body bashing' is usually more prevalent in males. This is the act of bashing one's body against a wall or even throwing oneself down the stairs. In some cases it may constitute bashing against somebody – for example, during team sports.

Self-harm of this kind can go undetected as falling down the stairs may be viewed as an accident. Bashing into someone and damaging a part of one's body during team sport may more often than not be passed off as an accident. These kind of recurring 'accidents' warrant attention.

Interfering with wound healing

In this case, the teenager purposefully and continuously hampers the healing of wounds by picking and over-rubbing. This can cause wounds to become infected.

Other forms of self-harm

Other forms of self-harm include:

- ✓ Substance misuse
- ✓ Alcohol abuse
- ✓ Over exercising
- ✓ Over eating
- ✓ Starving self
- ✓ Sexual promiscuity.

A study carried out by Whitlock *et al* (2006) examined the self-injurious behaviour of over 2800 college students. It found that 70% of those who repeatedly self-harmed reported engaging in two to four different self-harming methods. The findings of this study greatly correlate with my findings through working with teenagers who self-harm. Many in fact engage in hitting, scratching and pinching themselves when needing to deal with distress in more public places, like school, and will then engage in their preferred method – cutting, for example – when at home and alone in their room or bathroom later in the day.

Complications as a result of engaging in ongoing self-harm

Teenagers who engage in the act of self-harming do not usually intend to cause lasting injury. The purpose is to facilitate the release of stress, inducing an altered, more peaceful state, which in most cases is momentary, with feelings of guilt and shame emerging quickly.

Self-harming can lead to complications such as:

✓ Life-threatening blood loss through severing an artery
✓ Deep cuts which require stitching
✓ Scarring
✓ Breaking bones through body bashing
✓ Infections from interfering with wound healing or using dirty cutting objects
✓ Unintended suicide.

Prevalence of self-harm

The National Registry of Deliberate Self-Harm in Ireland (2012) recorded 12,010 presentations to hospital due to deliberate self-harm nationally, involving 9,483 individuals. Taking the population into account, the age-standardised rate of individuals presenting to hospital following deliberate self-harm in 2012 was 211 per 100,000. The rate of male presentation has increased by 20% since 2007 and the female rate increased by 6% over the same period. The most prevalent age range recorded for females was in the 15- to 19-year-old age group, at 617 per 100,000. The most prevalent age range among males was in the 20- to 24-year-old group, at 533 per 100,000. Drug overdose was the most common method of self-harm, presented at a rate of 69%; this method of self-harm was more common in females than males. Cutting accounted for 23% of presentations and was significantly more common in men than women.

The National Registry of Deliberate Self-harm in Northern Ireland West (2010) reported 1402 presentations to three Accident & Emergency and Urgent Care Departments in 2010, highlighting a 10.7% increase since 2009, 5.9% increase since 2008 and 2.4% increase since 2007. The highest rates of self-harm recorded were among those aged between 20 and 24 years, for both genders. Females represented a higher percentage of attendances, accounting for 55%. There were 102 attendances among those aged under 18 years, which accounted for 7.3% of all episodes. The majority of self-harm episodes presented by those aged under 18 years (68.6%) were female. Drug overdose was the predominant method of self-harm, particularly among females, accounting for 72.8% of all self-harm presentations. Self-cutting was the second most common form of self-harm, used in 18.4% of all self-harm presentations.

Research conducted by the Mental Health Foundation based in the UK found that the UK has one of the highest rates of self-harm in Europe, at 400 per 100,000 population. The South West Public Health Observatory (Cooke *et al* 2011), commissioned by NHS South West for commissioners and providers of health and social care, analysed data on suicide and self-harm in the South West and found that between 2001/02 and 2008/09 there were 68,136 self-harm admissions of residents aged 15 and over, with increasing rates in more recent years and with the fastest rises in young women aged 15-19 and 20-24 years.

Findings from the multicentre study of self-harm in England undertaken in six hospitals between 2000 and 2007 reported 7150 episodes of self-harm by 5205 individuals. In those aged 10-14 years, the rate averaged at 302 per 100,000 for girls, and 67 per 100,000 for boys, 'with a ratio of 5:1'. In those aged 15-17 years, the rates were 1,423 and 466, with a female:male ratio of 2.7:1. Of those presenting, over half had a history of self-harm. The most common type of self-harm was paracetamol overdose.

The Child and Adolescent Self-harm in Europe (CASE) Study (2005) concentrating on the responses of 30,000 15- to 16- year-olds to anonymous questionnaires, found that 70% of respondents admitted to self-harming at some stage in their lives (Madge *et al*, 2008).

Signs a teenager may be self-harming

Self-harming can be difficult to detect because of its secretive nature. The following signs may indicate that a teenager is self-harming:

✓ Looking for excuses not to engage in PE and sports activities like swimming
✓ Noticeable change in character
✓ Talking about him/herself in a negative way
✓ Unexplained wounds, scars and bruises
✓ Wearing long-sleeved tops and long trousers even in hot weather
✓ Disappearing more than usual and spending longer periods of time in his/her room, and locking the door
✓ More frequent and longer periods of time spent in the bathroom
✓ Lack of engagement with friends
✓ Noticeable collection of instruments that can cause injury and facilitate cutting
✓ A collection of plasters, soothing creams and antiseptics hidden in his/her room
✓ Blood spots on clothing and bed linen (turn clothes inside out to check)
✓ Refusing to go clothes shopping
✓ Finding laxatives in room, plus weight loss, and vomiting
✓ Reacting passively and retreating to room when challenged on an issue
✓ Looking for reasons to avoid family functions and seeking opportunities to be home alone more constantly and frequently.

What to do if you discover a teenager is self-harming

Discovering that a teenager is self-harming can be a daunting experience. You may feel afraid, angry and disgusted. On discovering a teenager is self-harming, action needs to be taken in a proactive rather than a reactive manner:

1. Attend to your own feelings; do not approach a teenager about your suspicions or observations until you are more relaxed and grounded.
2. Approach with compassion and understanding.
3. Time your approach; wait until you have the teenager alone and are sure you won't be interrupted.
4. Engage in a dialogue and outline your concerns in terms of what you have noticed. For example, 'Sarah, I wanted to have a chat with you. I have noticed that you are not yourself and I am worried about you.'
5. Now be direct: 'I have noticed that you have marks on your arm and I am wondering if you are self-harming.'
6. Do not get into a power struggle. The teenager will probably become defensive. Expect this reaction and remain composed and empathic.
7. Remember, the teenager will be struggling with his/her own feelings, which may include shame, anger and anxiety.
8. Keep dialogue going. Let the teenager know you are there to help, not judge, and that you appreciate this is difficult for them.
9. Outline what will happen next. For example, 'We will make an appointment with the doctor. We will find a therapist that will help you and I will support you all the way. We are in this together.'
10. If you are a professional who works with teenagers, you need to point out to the teenager that you have to

take action and inform the teenager's parents. This will no doubt be met with resistance. Remain composed and empathic and try your best to get the teenager to agree to such action. You have a duty of care and action needs to be taken to protect the welfare of the teenager. Refer to your agency's policies and procedures in relation to child protection and act accordingly.

11. If you are a parent who has discovered your child is self-harming, do not ignore what you have discovered. You may need to get emotional support yourself and I would advise that you engage with a service that can support you *and* your child. Services available are outlined in the Appendix (see page 133).

12. Listen, listen and listen! Do not get angry and judge; this will cause the teenager to close off from you and intensify his/her inner turmoil. Let him/her know you are aware of what is going on and appreciate he/she is in pain and you want to help.

13. Do not issue ultimatums in relation to stopping the self-harming behaviours. The act of self-harming is a coping mechanism and teenagers will not be able just simply to stop until the reasons for their actions have been uncovered and coping mechanisms that are more positive/nurturing have been developed through professional intervention.

14. Get professional help by engaging with a service that can support the teenager appropriately A list of services is available at the end of this book.

A very useful guide for parents and others is to 'AID' and 'ARM'. I explain these acronyms below. Keep them in mind when taking any action:

AID

A   Attend to your own feeling and compose yourself.

I   Inform the teenager you are aware of his/her self-harming with compassion and understanding.

D   Discuss the need for professional help and decide on appropriate actions together.

ARM

A   Activate a support system for yourself.

R   Refer the teenager for professional help and guidance.

M   Maintain a positive relationship with the teenager.

Alternative coping strategies

Through working with an experienced, empathic and compassionate professional many teenagers identity and utilise more nurturing coping methods to maintain their emotional and social wellbeing, moving from a place of self-harm to self-care. Coping mechanisms that are more nurturing and utilised by many of the teenagers I work with include:

✓   Keeping a diary and journaling their feelings

✓   Engaging in a physical activity, for example going for a walk or run, or swimming, depending on their interests and what they get pleasure and release from

✓   Connecting with a close friend who understands their struggles

✓   Talking with a supportive adult

✓   Ringing a help line

✓   Engaging in an art-and-craft activity

✓   Playing a musical instrument

✓   Breathing and relaxation techniques, such as mindfulness

✓   Caring for and soothing a pet

✓   Having a bath with relaxing aromatherapy oils

✓ Writing poetry

✓ Squeezing a stress ball; manipulating clay or play-dough.

The facts

✓ Self-harm is not necessarily an indication of suicide; it is a coping mechanism, utilised by many to stay alive.

✓ Self-harming is not attention seeking. It is a very secretive act and usually goes undetected for a long time. Teenagers who self-harm go to extreme lengths to hide their acts of self-harming and are usually uncovered by accident or through someone else noticing marks, scars or what appears to be ongoing accidental injury.

✓ It is incorrect to think only teenagers with a psychological disorder self-harm. While teenagers with mental health challenges may indeed engage in regular acts of self-harm, one does not have to have a psychological disorder to engage in this behviour. As previously stated, the act of self-harming is a coping mechanism used by teenagers as an emotional release from the distress and turmoil they are experiencing. Borderline Personality Disorder (BPD) is the only mental health disorder for which self-harm is a diagnostic feature. In my experience only a small minority of teenagers who self-harm meet the diagnostic criteria for this condition. Self-harming behaviour alone should never result in the assumption that a person has BPD. BPD should and can only be diagnosed following a comprehensive assessment by a psychologist or psychiatrist.

Self-Harm Intervention Skills Training – STORM (www.stormskillstraining.com)

STORM® began as a research project at the University of

Manchester, UK, in the 1990s as a response to the need for training in specific skills-based self-harm risk assessment and management. Research has found that this training programme increases skills, improves attitudes to self-harming and improves confidence in assessing risk and safety planning. It consists of:

Module 1: Self-injury risk assessment – Assessing self-injury: preceding events, current intention and seriousness; physical assessment of injury.

Module 2: Crisis management – Ensuring safety; building a network of support; identifying copying mechanisms and strategies.

Module 3: Problem solving – Brief self-help technique to teach clients in a crisis.

STORM® Self Injury Training gives frontline workers the necessary skills for assessing and managing self-injury among their client group. The training explores attitudes to self-injury, the relationship of self-injury to suicide, emotional and psychological states in lead up to a crisis, skills in harm minimisation and the development of alternative coping strategies.

Chapter summary – Self-harm

Self-harm has an enormous effect on the lives of teenagers who utilise this flawed mechanism to cope with their distress. The act is secretive and repetitive. The burden of self-harm can be hard to carry, as can the guilt and shame associated with the act. A vicious cycle emerges and many have no clue how to break the cycle, which can result in the acts of self-harming becoming more frequent and progressive in nature. We must remember that the act of self-harming is serving a purpose, relieving stress momentarily. Recovery is not as simple as just stopping. In the majority of cases, self-harming does dissipate and cease only when teenagers have developed and embraced more effective and nurturing ways of coping with their distress. This will be explored in more detail in Chapter 4, Talk therapies (see page 49). All behaviour has a function and purpose. The key to supporting a teenager who engages in self-harming acts is to uncover the reasons for these behaviours.

Chapter 3

Suicide
– the fatal consequence of 'self-defeatist syndrome'

Suicide is a permanent solution to a temporary problem.

Phil Donohue

Suicide is misunderstood and often associated with those who have a mental illness. Research informs us that people who have a mental illness are more prone to suicidal ideation (thinking) and some unfortunately complete suicide. However, an increasing number of teenagers are taking their own lives not as a result of a mental health issue but because of a crisis they are ill equipped to deal with, and as such the option of suicide becomes very inviting. According to the World Health Organisation, almost one million people die by suicide each year worldwide, representing an annual global suicide mortality rate of 16 per 100,000. Suicide is the second leading cause of death among 15- to 29-year-olds. Ireland has the fourth highest rate of youth suicide in the expanded EU, after Lithuania, Finland and Estonia, at 15.7 per 100,000 for 15-24 year olds. Suicide is a leading cause of death in Scotland among people aged 15-34 years. In the United Kingdom, 6045, 5608 and 5675 people aged 15 and over died by suicide in 2011, 2010 and 2009 respectively. These statistics are alarming to say the least. We need to understand and become aware of the many reasons why a teenager might consider and complete suicide. In doing so we will be enabled to deal with the issue in a proactive manner and offer the much needed support that people in an emotional crisis need.

Myths about suicide

✓ A teenager who talks about ending his/her life is looking for attention –

A teenager who talks or makes reference to taking his/her own life is in need of attention and his/her statements and references to dying need and must be taken seriously. He/she is clearly in distress and vulnerable and needs immediate attention, support and intervention.

✓ Talking to and asking a teenager if he/she is suicidal will encourage him/her to complete suicide –

Talking about suicide is a positive step. Opening a dialogue with a teenager you are concerned about will not encourage that person to take his/her life but may well encourage him/her to stay alive. Talking about suicide with distressed teenagers will enable them to express their feelings and feel supported, and with the right professional interventions they will be enabled to resolve the issues that are causing them distress and move to a more positive place.

✓ Teenagers who make a suicide attempt or complete suicide have a mental illness –

Some teenagers with a mental health diagnosis may be more susceptible to suicidal thinking and completion. However, many teenagers who do not have a mental health issue contemplate and complete suicide as a result of an emotional crisis they are ill equipped to deal with, coupled with a lack of support.

✓ A teenager who plans his/her suicide cannot be stopped – A teenager who has a suicide plan is at a greater risk as he/she has given thought to his/her death and has planned how it will be carried out. A teenager who has an *active* plan needs to have this plan disarmed; immediate professional intervention is warranted. A teenager who had planned to take his/her own life does not want to die. He/she is so distressed and in so much pain, ending his/her life appears the only way to make the pain stop. Helping a teenager deal with his/her pain will enable him/her to heal and move to a better place over time.

Youth suicide risk factors

The probability of a teenager contemplating and completing suicide depends on the interplay of multiple factors. The risk of suicide is significantly increased when a teenager struggles with several of the risk factors outlined here, at the same time.

A recent significant loss

Experiencing a loss can have a profound effect on a person's wellbeing. All that was secure, safe and familiar no longer exists. This can be extremely painful and daunting for a teenager to navigate and comprehend.

The death of a loved family member or friend
Losing someone we have a strong emotional attachment to can be very distressing. The pain and anguish caused by the death of a loved one can be engulfing and unfamiliar. A sense of panic, isolation and hopelessness can distort a teenager's thinking and logic, bringing him/her to a dark scary place where suicide is contemplated. Teenagers who have experienced a loss through the death of a loved one need to be held and supported; they

need to be guided, listened to and understood. They need the time and space to talk about their loss and have their feelings validated and normalised. In my experience, the power of an empathic listening ear can help move a teenager from a place of anguish, distress and isolation to a place of reorientation and acceptance, in time. In instances where teenagers present with suicidal thinking as a result of a significant loss, I believe that it is vital not only to listen to, and validate, their feelings but also to spend time explaining the grieving process and normaling their feelings. This in turn can help to lift their suicidal thinking and assist them in uncovering reasons for living while continuing healthy bonds with their deceased loved one.

A relationship break-up with a boyfriend or girlfriend

Relationships with peers are very important to teenagers and a key part of their developmental process. During the teenager years, as we all know, romantic relationships develop; some blossom into something special while others end without mutual agreement, causing a great level of upset and feelings of rejection. A myriad of feelings emerges that are unfamiliar and painful; these feeling can affect teenagers' mental wellbeing, causing them to doubt their worth, their sense of self and their place amongst their peer group.

The ending of a romantic relationship can plunge a teenager into despair and lead to the onset of self-harming, suicidal ideation and, unfortunately for some, suicide. These feelings of rejection and being unloved by someone they love dearly can be all too painful for some teenagers to navigate. Many teenagers can feel a great sense of displacement, shame, anger and rejection when the person they love ends the relationship; these feelings are totally understandable – nobody likes to be dumped! Some teenagers are well equipped to manage and work through a break-up, but for some it can be too much to handle, particularly if they have low self-esteem and no support systems.

Chapter 3

In cases where teenagers present with suicidal ideation or self-harming as a result of a break-up, professionals need to listen attentively and explore what the relationship was like, uncovering what needs were being met by the relationship, bearing in mind it may have had an unhealthy foundation. What I mean by an unhealthy foundation is the seeking of another's love and approval to fill a void or sense of inadequacy within oneself. In my experience, many teenagers who exhibit suicidal thoughts, self-harming or a suicide attempt as a result of a relationship break-up have deeper issues at play. For many, they are not aware of these underlying issues or unmet needs as these feelings are more often than not suppressed and filed away in the teenager's subconscious mind as they are too painful to acknowledge and express. These unmet needs from the past need to be uncovered and addressed gently and slowly with the help of a skilled professional, ensuring supports are put in place in order to build the teenager's resilience, self-compassion and self-esteem.

Parental separation

Parental separation can affect teenagers in many different ways, depending on how the separation is managed. Some teenagers may experience a range of emotions when their parents separate, including relief, confusion, self-blame, anger, shame, resentment, rejection, fear, loss, sadness and uncertainty about the future. It can be a very daunting time for teenagers and as a result of this many may resort to self-harming or contemplate suicide to escape the emotional turmoil and overwhelming feelings they are experiencing. In my experience many teenagers can feel so overwhelmed by their parents' separation that they suppress their feelings as they do not want to cause their parents any more stress and anxiety.

Having a place to come to where they can express their feelings and voice their concerns with a compassionate adult can help move a teenager to a more balanced place in a short period of time. In my work supporting teenagers whose parents have separated, many report being concerned about the future and have questions they would like answered but are generally afraid to ask their parents for fear of upsetting them. In this situation, I facilitate teenagers in expressing their concerns while also exploring what outcomes they would like and how they can express these needs and desires to their parents. I have found this approach to be highly beneficial and empowering. In most cases, once these concerns and questions have been answered, and new consistent routines established, self-harming and suicidal thoughts do diminish very quickly.

Moving to a new location

Moving to a new place that is not familiar can cause a teenager to become distressed and apprehensive. Peers and friends are a central element in a teenager's life and the prospect of being separated from friends and moving to a new location and a new school can be very unnerving. The thought of losing connections with their peer group and moving to a new school can be too much to bear for some teenagers and as a result they may engage in self-harming and have suicidal thoughts, as moving away from friends can seem like the end of their world.

In situations where a move is planned, I would strongly recommend that teenagers are consulted and involved in the process. They need to be given the space and time to air their concerns and have their feelings validated and appreciated. A teenager who is struggling with a move to a new location needs to be supported, and parents are advised to be alert and mindful of the effects that leaving friends behind can have on a teenager. Support systems need to be put in place to make the transition easier and every effort must be made to enable the teenager to maintain links with close friends. Parents are advised to speak to school personnel and inform them that their teenager is finding the transition difficult; this will ensure the school takes an empathic view towards the teenager and supports him/her in the transition.

Teenagers' hobbies and interests need to be supported; I would strongly advise that parents encourage their teenagers to join community groups related to those interests so they can develop new friendships and prevent isolation.

Parents need to be mindful that their teenager is navigating his/her way through the unknown; this can be very daunting as all that was familiar is no longer present. A great level of uncertainty and fear can cause teenagers to regress and bring them to a dark place. With support and encouragement, teenagers generally do settle into their new environment within a couple of months. However, parents need to be patient and empathic, and ensure community participation while keeping the lines of communication open.

Rejection by peers

During the adolescent years, friends become the cornerstone of teenagers' lives; friends are vital and a valuable support system. When this system breaks down and the teenager feels rejected and isolated, thoughts of suicide and acts of self-harm can emerge. Being rejected by a friend and peer group can be soul destroying for a teenager and can have a knock-on effect in so many other areas of a teenager's life; in my experience many find attending school difficult; many stop going to their social outlets, like dance classes or training sessions, thus compounding their sense of isolation even more. Anxiety levels soar and their self-esteem becomes compromised, leading to thoughts of suicide and engaging in acts of self-harming to release inner pain.

In this situation, the teenager needs to be handled with care, understanding and compassion. It is vital to spend time hearing his/her story and building his/her self-esteem. It is also vital to move him/her from ruminating about the issue to a solution-focused stance where problems are aired and a range of solutions explored and implemented which the teenager is comfortable with. What is key in this situation is for the teenager's story to be heard and his/her feelings validated while he/she is helped to discover and implement workable solutions to the issue that meet his/her needs and wishes.

Prior suicide attempt

A prior suicide attempt is a significant risk factor for a teenager making another suicide attempt, and for completing suicide, if the reasons for the first attempt have not been uncovered and dealt with in a timely, compassionate manner, with a skilled professional. Approximately 20% of people who die by suicide have made a prior suicide attempt; research informs us that the risk of completing suicide is elevated during the days and weeks following hospitalisation for a suicide attempt. After a teenager has been discharged from A&E or from hospital after a suicide attempt, great care needs to be taken to ensure his/her recovery and ongoing wellbeing.

The issue of teenagers completing suicide after being discharged from A&E departments and after a period of hospitalisation is well documented in the media. Many are discharged still in the midst of a crisis, with no support systems in place; this is totally unacceptable but unfortunately in some cases a reality.

I strongly advise that family members ensure support systems are in place for their loved one and, indeed, for themselves. It is advisable that family members caring for a loved one who has made a suicide attempt take a proactive approach to ensure their loved one receives the care and support they need during this challenging time. The teenager who has made a suicide attempt needs professional help and should be encouraged to seek counselling and the assistance of support groups and community engagement.

If a teenager has been prescribed medication, parents are advised to take control of this as leaving this to the teenager is inviting trouble, especially if he/she is still feeling low, despondent and suicidal.

Parents need to be extra diligent during this period. A teenager still in the midst of a crisis is vulnerable and should not be left alone or with access to any means that could enable self-harm – or suicide. The person in distress cannot heal in isolation, and family members need direction and support on how to manage their loved one and themselves during this challenging period. A list of support services is outlined in the Appendix (see page 133).

Death of a family member or friend through suicide

Exposure to completed and attempted suicide in one's family and peer group has been found to increase suicide risk among vulnerable teenagers. Losing a loved one through suicide does not necessarily mean that a teenager will contemplate or complete suicide; however, although rare, experiencing such a traumatic loss can be a risk factor.

Grief is a complicated and individual process and affects people in many different ways. Losing someone dear to suicide is very distressing and the feelings that emerge can be complicated and exhausting to deal with. Teenagers can have a difficult time dealing with these feelings and the grieving process. Those who lose a friend or family member through suicide need to be handled with compassion, but also be given a clear message that suicide is not something to romanticise.

All too often, social networking sites do inadvertently romanticise suicide, which can spark vulnerable, distressed teenagers into making impulsive decisions with devastating consequences. There has been a lot of coverage in the press over the last number of years in relation to teen copycat and cluster suicides. We need to reframe the romanticising of suicide, particularly for vulnerable, distressed and impulsive teenagers, giving a clear message that suicide is not the answer.

It is vital that schools, parents, youth leaders and those who support and work with teenagers handle a loss through suicide with sensitivity and compassion, while also giving a clear message that help and support are available and sign-post teenagers in the right direction so they may receive appropriate support and interventions.

Abuse

Sexual abuse and, to a lesser extent, physical abuse, in childhood have proved to be a risk factor for suicidal ideation, suicide attempts and, unfortunately, suicide completion. Sexual abuse spans the spectrum of all forms of abuse as it incorporates physical abuse, emotional abuse and neglect.

Experiencing abuse as a child can have a marked effect on a person's wellbeing. Teenager who have suffered ongoing abuse, particularly sexual abuse, can experience a great sense of powerlessness, shame, guilt, isolation and self-loathing, which can have a negative impact on their psychological functioning and lead them to a place where suicide is contemplated.

The impact of abuse on a teenager's wellbeing is more severely compromised when:

- ✓ The abuse experienced was ongoing and frequent.
- ✓ A high level of physical force was applied.
- ✓ The perpetrator was someone who was trusted and well regarded by the victim.

Research informs us that continual sexual abuse is a major risk factor and strongly associated with suicide attempts, more so than a single occurrence. Sexual abuse by an immediate family carries the highest risk.

Specialised intervention by a qualified professional is warranted if a disclosure of sexual abuse has been made by a teenager. The effectiveness of treatment and recovery is enhanced when the teenager who has experienced abuse is believed and supported by their family. Family cohesion is especially important for helping teenagers affected by child sexual abuse to cope with their experiences and reclaim control over their lives.

Support and intervention by a qualified professional can help teenagers by:

✓ Reducing feelings of anger, shame, and guilt surrounding the abuse

✓ Enhancing their self-image and self esteem

✓ Developing nurturing coping-mechanisms

✓ Moving from a place of victim to survivor.

Recovery from abuse can and does happen. The entire family is affected by abuse, particularly sexual abuse, and, therefore, recovery is improved and sustained when family members are involved and engage in the treatment process.

If a teenager discloses any form of abuse, action needs to be taken in a timely manner to protect the welfare of the teenager and of others who may be at risk from the perpetrator. We are now in an era where the needs and the interests of children have become a priority. Child protection legislation has gone some way to ensuring that children are protected and receive appropriate support. This is a welcome development.

All agencies and services that work with and support under 18s must have child protection policies and procedures for staff to follow and implement. If a teenager discloses any form of abuse, as a professional one has a duty of care to the teenager and the wider community and must act accordingly. If you are such a professional, you must refer to and become familiar with your agency's policies and procedures on child protection and follow them, ensuring guidance and support from your agency's child protection officer. Abuse can be a complex, difficult and frightening situation to deal with; however, the welfare of the teenager who has made a disclosure is of paramount importance.

Sexual orientation

The teenage years are a time in which young people develop their identity and autonomy. During this developmental stage, teenagers gradually become more aware of themselves as sexual beings, developing interests and desires. The development of adolescent sexuality spans the physical, cognitive, emotional and social domains. During this period teenagers commonly begin to identify themselves as being:

- ✓   Heterosexual – attracted to members of the opposite sex
- ✓   Homosexual – attracted to members of the same sex
- ✓   Bisexual – attracted to members of both sexes.

For many this is an exciting period, but for others it can be a time of great distress and uncertainty. Struggling with one's sexual identity and orientation has been highlighted as a risk factor for teenage suicidal ideation and completion in recent years. Gay and lesbian adults often describe their teenage years as a time in which they felt isolated, lonely and afraid due to narrow societal views. It has been reported in many research papers that victimisation may be a leading factor in the high rates of suicidal thinking and completion in this population.

Societal views and expectations can have a profound effect on teenagers' wellbeing, particularly if those teenagers are judged, isolated and rejected because of their sexual orientation, which for some unfortunately is a very real, lived experience.

Bullying

Bullying can be a catalyst for considering, attempting and completing suicide. Its significance should never be overlooked. The detrimental effects ongoing bullying can have on the social and emotional wellbeing of teenagers have been widely reported in the media over recent years. Many unfortunately feel ill-equipped to deal with the anguish bullying causes; life for many becomes a struggle, with thoughts of suicide becoming ever more inviting. In the pre-internet era, much bullying was limited to school hours, but these days, modern technology facilitates it to continue at all times, penetrating all elements of the teenager's life and environment.

Bullying can take many forms, from being made fun of and degraded in front of others, to name calling and being the subject of vicious and untrue rumours; from being threatened with and experiencing physical harm to being pressurised to steal and give money to the perpetuators; from being excluded from activities and events on purpose, to having property vandalised. The issue of bullying must never go unaddressed as the consequences can prove fatal.

Drug and alcohol misuse

Drug and alcohol abuse can cause great distress, leading to social isolation, low self-esteem, loss of work or school, and estrangement from family and friends – all events that can build a core of stresses that may lead to suicidal thoughts and completion. Substance abuse also can increase impulsiveness and decrease inhibitions, making the teenager more likely to act on suicidal thoughts.

Signs a teenager may be contemplating suicide

✓   Speaking a lot about suicide or death in a positive

or romanticised manner, particularly if someone the teenager has respected and admired completed suicide.

✓ Writing about death or drawing pictures depicting death.

✓ Researching death on the internet and ways of dying (check internet history).

✓ Posting stressful messages and comments about death and dying on social media.

✓ Making statements like: 'I'd be better off dead', 'You would all be better off without me', 'I can't cope with this anymore', 'You won't have to worry about me for much longer', 'I wish I had never been born'.

✓ Making ongoing comments about being hopeless, helpless or worthless.

✓ Giving away possessions that mean a lot to the teenager to people they care about.

✓ Changes in personality – for example, a teenager who was once happy and easy-going becoming angry and hostile.

✓ Changes in eating patterns – for example, over-eating for emotional comfort or losing interest in eating.

✓ Changes in sleeping patterns – for example, over-sleeping or being unable to sleep; ongoing wakefulness and interrupted sleep.

✓ Unprovoked bouts of crying.

✓ Neglecting personal appearance and hygiene.

✓ Lack of interest in activities the teenager previously enjoyed and derived pleasure from.

✓ Significant decrease in school performance and a lack of motivation around attending school and completing school work.

✓ Starting to abuse drugs or alcohol as a means to escape from inner turmoil.

✓ Isolation – withdrawing from family members and

friends, spending more and more time alone, not answering the phone, not returning missed calls and turning off his/her mobile for long periods of time without due reason.

✓ Acting on impulse with no thought or fear to the consequences of their actions.

✓ Saying goodbye to family and friends in a way that indicates they may not see them again.

✓ Suddenly appearing very cheerful, content and at ease after a long period of appearing down, isolated and disinterested. This is a key warning sign that is often missed and mistaken as a teenager being back to his/her own self. However, this may be an indication that the teenager has planned his/her suicide and has come to terms with ending his/her life, and as a result feels a great sense of relief and contentment around the decision to die.

Be alert to the following three Hs:

✓ **Hopelessness** – Teenagers appear in a state of despair with the inability to see any hope and resolution to their problems.

✓ **Haplessness** – Teenagers show no interest and derive little pleasure from activities and interactions they previously enjoyed and valued.

✓ **Helplessness** – Teenagers appear lost, despondent and isolated, indicating that nothing can or will help them.

What to do if you are concerned about a teenager's wellbeing

If you are concerned about a teenager's wellbeing, I recommend you employ what is termed a **FRIEND-TER-VENTION** using the following guidelines:

STOP

S   Seek out the teenager you are concerned about and sit with them.

T   Talk to them about your concerns for their welfare and your observations.

O   Open up a dialogue about how they are feeling, their thoughts and any plans.

P   Plan together for professional help. Ensuring the teenagers is linked in with a skilled professional will ensure their concerns and problems are dealt with and resolved appropriately.

HOPE

H   Help by:

O   Opening up lines of communication.

P   Planning for professional interventions.

E   Ensuring engagement with professional services.

Applied Suicide Intervention Skills Training – ASIST (www.livingworks.net)

ASIST trains participants to reduce the immediate risk of a suicide and increase support for the person at risk. This programme affords participants the opportunity to gain an understanding of what a person at risk may need from them in order to keep safe. This programme encourages honest, open and direct talk about suicide as part of preparing participants to provide suicide first aid. Participants will also explore how personal attitudes and experiences might affect their helping role with a person at risk of suicide.

On completion, participants will be enabled to:

✓ recognise invitations to help
✓ reach out and offer support
✓ review the risk of suicide
✓ develop a safety plan
✓ link with community resources.

Chapter summary – Suicide

Suicide is a major concern in today's society, with an increasing number of young people dying by suicide internationally. Suicidal thoughts, attempts and completion are more heightened and likely when a teenager's psychological, environmental and social needs are not met. The more risk factors a teenager experiences and is exposed to, the greater the risk. A teenager who makes any kind of reference to taking his/her own life must be taken seriously and appropriate interventions and professional help sought in a timely manner. Employ a **FRIEND-TER-VENTION**: **STOP** and give **HOPE**.

Chapter 4

Talk therapies

Each time you're kind, gentle, and encouraging, each time you try to understand because you really care, my heart begins to grow wings.

Charles C. Finn

This chapter will introduce you to the main 'talk therapies' used by skilled and experienced professionals that have been proven to be effective in helping teenagers overcome their problems and restore inner harmony and self-esteem. Many of the strategies outlined can also be utilised by parents and other professionals.

'Talk therapies' is the umbrella term used to describe a range of therapeutic interventions based on talking through and exploring solutions to problems with a trained professional. There are many models, techniques and interventions applied, and advocated, by many different schools of thought, each having the ultimate goal of assisting clients to heal and develop.

Understanding the role of different professionals

Counsellor

A counsellor will generally work with clients for a short period of time, facilitating and encouraging behavioural change in the here and now. A counsellor assists clients in identifying problems, supports them in times of crisis and encourages them to take positive steps to resolve their issues and concerns, with a focus on a more positive future.

Psychotherapist

A psychotherapist usually works with clients over a longer period of time, focusing on and exploring a client's past experiences, thus facilitating clients to gain a deeper awareness of their emotional issues and their sources. Unresolved issues and traumas are explored and confronted, with the ultimate aim being to come to terms with these issues, facilitating client healing and the development of new awareness.

Psychiatrist

A psychiatrist is a medical doctor who specialises in the assessment, diagnosis, treatment, and prevention of mental health and emotional difficulties. A psychiatrist will offer advice, and recommend different treatments including medication, counselling, psychotherapy or other lifestyle interventions that best suit the client and the condition he/she is presenting with.

Psychologist

A psychologist is a trained professional whose role is to reduce psychological distress and enhance and promote the psychological wellbeing of clients through assessment, diagnosis, treatment planning and support. Psychologists are not licensed to prescribe medication; only psychiatrists and other medical doctors may do so.

Chapter 4

Main tenets of all models of talk therapy

Every therapeutic relationship should have at its core the principles of empathy, unconditional positive regard and congruence. These key therapeutic principals were set out and advocated by Carl Rogers (1902-1987) in his model of therapy called 'person-centred therapy'.

Empathy is best described as the ability to step into another person's shoes, thus becoming aware, appreciative and mindful of their lived experience. This is facilitated by actively listening and appreciating the experience from the client's point of view, truly understanding and accepting his/her feelings. This is a key skill in building a positive and engaging relationship.

Unconditional positive regard – In demonstrating 'unconditional positive regard' towards a client, a mental health professional ensures there are no conditions placed on acceptance; he/she displays a non-judgemental attitude towards the client in which the client feels supported, respected and valued as a person.

Congruence – In operating with 'congruence', a mental health professional will not hide behind his/her professional stance but will demonstrate that he/she too is human. Congruence is demonstrated through being genuinely interested, open and transparent, and is integral to all interactions with clients.

These three elements are the foundation of any therapeutic relationship. In my professional experience, teenagers need to feel appreciated, understood and supported if they are to engage and share the challenges they are experiencing. Ensuring these three elements are demonstrated will ultimately set the stage for engagement and the development of a teenager's wellbeing and resilience.

Key models of intervention

Solution-focused brief therapy

Solution-focused brief therapy (SFBT), also known as 'solution focused therapy', was developed by Steve de Shazer (1940-2005) and Insoo Kim Berg (1934-2007), and their colleagues, in the late 1970s at the Brief Family Therapy Centre of Milwaukee, Wisconsin, USA. SFBT is a short-term, goal-focused therapeutic model which focuses on solutions to problems, rather than on the problems themselves, while remaining empathic towards the client and the distress he/she is experiencing.

The therapist's goal is to encourage and motivate teenagers to envisage their future as they would like it to be, collaboratively working together in developing a series of steps and tasks to help and empower them to achieve their desired goals. The therapist works with teenagers to help them uncover and realise their hidden, unacknowledged, suppressed skills and resources. This model validates strengths and empowers teenagers to realise that they have power and control over their current situation

JS Kim and C Franklin (2009) reviewed literature in relation to the benefits of employing 'a solution-focused brief therapy model' in a school setting. This review found SFBT to be particularly effective in reducing the intensity of negative feelings and the management of behavioural problems in school-age populations.

Main tenets of SFBT
The main tenets of SFBT are:

- ✓ Short-term intervention
- ✓ Change is continual and to be anticipated
- ✓ Clients are regarded as experts in their own lives with a wealth of knowledge
- ✓ Clients are encouraged to identify and develop their life goals and desires

✓   Goals can be achieved once broken down into small steps

✓   Clients become aware of what is possible, achievable and viable for them to accomplish when validated and motivated

✓   Past problems do not define the client

✓   Clients have control in the here and now

✓   One small change can have a domino effect.

It is vital that the therapist:

1. Ascertains and uncovers the teenager's goals for therapy and hopes for the future.
2. Encourages and motivates the teenager to visualise what his/her life would be like if these hopes and goals were achieved.
3. Assists the teenager to reflect and realise what he/she can do, or may be unaware that he/she is currently doing, to achieve these goals.
4. Compliments and validates all achievements no matter how small they may be.

SFBT techniques

Coping questions

Coping questions are used to uncover and validate how a teenager has managed his/her concerns, issues and problems to date. I have found that employing this technique aids teenagers in becoming aware of their coping skills and that they are managing at some level. Inviting them to share how they have coped to date helps to uncover existing skills and resources they have utilised and provides a foundation upon which to build further solutions.

Key questions I generally ask include:

How have you coped with this situation before you came to see me?

What has helped you to keep going?

Who did you seek out for support?

What did they do that was helpful?

What do you do that stops the problem getting worse?

What else?

Exceptions

While a teenager may initially appear hopeless and helpless about his/her current situation, the SFBT therapist must uncover exceptions to the problems presented. This is facilitated by uncovering and challenging the teenager to think of times when the problem was not so powerful and overwhelming. Uncovering and acknowledging that there are and were times in which the problem was less intense and manageable in my experience facilitates the teenager in realising that problems can be overcome and managed and can give a great sense of empowerment and hope. This aids a shift in thinking from problem-focused to solution-orientated, which is a valuable life skill.

Key questions I ask include:

Have you noticed anything being better since our last appointment? What is different? What is better?

Can you think of a time when you did not have this problem?

What would have to happen for you to feel positive again?

Can you remember when the problem did not take over and you felt okay?

What was different about those times?

Let's think about what you were doing or thinking that was different and more helpful during those better times?

What have you been doing more of that you find helpful?

What else?

Scaling questions

Scaling questions are used to help and empower teenagers to assess their own situation and track their progress and levels of motivation. I have found utilising scaling questions to be a key strategy in monitoring progress towards a goal, levels of confidence, and commitment to achieving a desired goal.

Examples of scaling questions I often use include:

On a scale of 1 to 10, where 10 is really good and positive and 1 is very low and negative, how are you today?

On a scale of 1 to 10, with 10 meaning you feel you have gained control over the problems and 1 meaning the problem is still controlling you, where would you rate your progress?

If 10 means you are extremely motivated to find solutions and 1 means you have no motivation at all, where would you place your levels of motivation?

You have identified yourself as being at 4, which is an improvement; well done! Now what do we need to do to move you to 5?

Miracle question

In asking teenagers the miracle question they are invited to imagine and brainstorm possibilities, changes they would like and how achieving those changes would feel. This is a very powerful technique and extremely motivating. I have found that asking the miracle question opens up a range of possibilities and solutions that the teenager may have never thought of before and is very empowering and motivational.

Examples of miracle questions I tend to ask include:

Suppose you had a magic wand and this wand would change your situation, what would be different?

Just imagine I had a crystal ball in which you could see that your problem was no longer present. What would your life look like?

If your wish was granted, what would your life be like without this problem?

The miracle question encourages teenagers to imagine possibilities and thus facilitates the development of solutions in order to achieve their miracle. I have found that the following questions help to move teenagers into action in terms of achieving their goal:

What would you be doing differently?

What would other people notice about you?

What would you notice about yourself?

What can we plan today to help you take one step closer? (This is a key question for empowering teenagers to take action.)

Compliments

Complimenting coping skills, motivation and achievements is a very important factor within the SFBT model. Complimenting teenagers on their success, no matter how small, reinforces capabilities and strengths. I utilise compliments in all sessions, making sure I am extremely attentive to changes, progress, efforts and developments observed. I spend time drawing teenagers' attention to my observations of their progress no matter how small; this I have found aids the development of self-esteem and confidence.

Plan

All sessions should end with a plan. What will the teenager do until their next session that will take him/her a step closer to achieving his/her goal? This is important as teenagers need to be challenged and motivated to help themselves. If they do not achieve their goal this needs to be discussed at the next session and further supports developed and put in place to enable them to do so.

SFBT therapists consistently remind and encourage clients to remember tomorrow and not the problems of the past, focusing on what is and can be more positive in their lives.

Cognitive behavioural therapy (CBT)

Cognitive behavioural therapy (CBT) was developed by Dr Aaron Beck in the 1960s, while he was a psychiatrist at the University of Pennsylvania. CBT is a structured, time-limited intervention which is goal orientated and educative, with a focus on relapse prevention.

Kaslow and Thompson (1998) and Kazdin and Weisz (1998) produced literature reviews that determined that CBT was an effective treatment model for depressed teenagers, highlighting that this treatment model demonstrated positive outcomes which were scientifically sound and valid.

CBT is based on the concept that how we think (that is, our cognition) affects how we feel our emotions and this in turn causes us to act, react and behave in certain ways. Simply put, our thoughts influence our feelings and our feelings influence our behaviours.

The model can be formulated as follows:

Activating event – The event or situation that triggers the teenager's automatic negative thoughts.

Beliefs – The teenager's beliefs and interpretation of the event or situation, which are usually negative and irrational

Consequences – The teenager's feelings, thoughts and actions as a result of their irrational thoughts about the situation or event.

CBT therapists uncover and challenge cognitive distortions and facilitate teenagers to think about their thought processes, feelings and actions in a healthier fashion. A teenager in the midst of what I call 'self-defeating syndrome' will more often than not present to the CBT therapist with the following cognitive distortions, which need to be challenged for change to occur:

Catastrophising means automatically anticipating the worst possible outcome will occur (for example, 'There is no point in trying to study for my exams. I am way behind and won't pass anyway.').

Filtering means amplifying the negative and minimising the positive aspects of an experience. The-glass-is-half-empty, opposed to half-full thinking. (for example, 'My friend called around. He only called on me because he had nothing else to do and the rest of the lads were busy.').

Personalising means automatically believing you are responsible for a negative or unpleasant event, where there is little or no proof for drawing this conclusion (for example, 'My friend said he would call me yesterday after lunch but he never did. He just said he would, but I knew he wouldn't because he thinks I'm a fool and boring.'). It may be that the friend in question actually was unable to call for a very valid reason.

Over-generalising means viewing an isolated negative experience as an absolute (for example, 'John dumped me because I'm a geek. No one will ever want to go out with me. I will never have a chance of a happy relationship.').

Black or white/polarised thinking refers to an all-or-nothing view of situations, with no middle ground. There is no room for reasoning or looking for possibilities. (for example, 'I rang Jack. He never rang back. He doesn't care about me. He has started to hang out with John, his new friend, now. If Jack was my friend he would just want to hang out with me.').

Emotional reasoning refers to allowing feelings to supersede logical evaluation of the event or situation. Feelings are viewed as facts (for example, 'I feel so hopeless. That means the situation is hopeless and can't be remedied.').

Mind reading refers to the assumption that people are reacting to you in a negative way, with no proof (for example, 'I walked into my maths class and the lads were laughing at me.'). The fact may be that the teenager's friends were telling a joke and having a laugh over it just as he/she walked in.

The role of the CBT therapist is to support teenagers while actively challenging their negative automatic thoughts and beliefs for validity and also educating them on how these thought patterns link to self-defeating behaviours.

Cognitive behavioural techniques
Socratic questioning

The function of 'Socratic questioning' (so-called after the Ancient Greek philosopher, who approached philosophical issues in this way) is to encourage and facilitate teenagers in becoming more self-aware by challenging the validity and accuracy of their belief systems, and exposing their cognitive distortions, thus helping them to realise that their current thinking is self-defeatist and unproductive.

Examples of clarifying questions I use include:

What do you mean when you say ...?

Could you explain a bit more about that?

What is the main point you are making?

Could you share an example?

Could you put that another way?

What I am hearing you say is ..., is that correct?

The last question communicates to teenagers that you are listening and want to understand how they are thinking and feeling. It also gives teenagers the opportunity to correct you if you have misinterpreted what they are trying to convey.

Examples of assumption questions I use include:

What you are assuming here is ...? Is that correct?

How have you rationalised this to be true?

Is this always the case?

What do you think the assumption holds here?

Why would someone make that assumption?

Examples of evidence and reason questions, which are key to challenging distortions in thinking, include:

How do you know this for sure?

Is there any reason to doubt this?

Do you have any concrete evidence?

Could you share your reasons for thinking this?

How could we find out if this is correct?

This last question helps teenagers to come up with solutions and other options.

Examples of origin and sources questions that I use include:

Have you always felt this way?

What causes you to feel this way? [Triggers!]

Where did you get this idea from?

Do your friends feel the same way? How do you know?

Do your family feel the same way? How do you know?

Examples of implications and consequences questions I find helpful are:

If you were to do that, what might that suggest to your mother/father/friend/ teacher etc?

When you say ..., are you suggesting that ...?

If you took that option, what could this lead to?

What effect would this action have? (This question helps the teenager consider consequences, be they positive or negative. If action would have a negative effect, then more time needs to be given to explore more positive actions.)

Is there another alternative?

Examples of viewpoint and perspective questions that I find helpful are:

How would your dad/mum/friend/teacher/coach respond? Why do you think she/he would respond in this way?

Could you share why this is necessary or beneficial? Who would benefit?

What would someone who disagrees with you say?

Is there an alternative?

Homework
Homework is a key element of the CBT model. Teenagers are encouraged to complete homework tasks between sessions in order to facilitate and promote cognitive restructuring. Homework encourages teenagers to practise and utilise skills learned during sessions, monitor and challenge their automatic negative thoughts, review the previous therapy session, and prepare for the next therapy session. Homework assignments include charting thoughts, feelings and behaviours in order to challenge negative thinking and foster healthier ways of thinking; practising soothing techniques such as relaxation and visual imagery; and recording positive affirmations in a journal.

Key tenets of CBT
The CBT therapist must:

- ✓ Identify and challenge the teenager's automatic negative thoughts.
- ✓ Encourage and challenge the teenager to actively engage in satisfying, mood-boosting activities.
- ✓ Encourage the teenager to engage in social connections.
- ✓ Develop and enhance problem-solving competences.
- ✓ Facilitate and educate the teenager on how to decrease physiological tension.

The ultimate goal of CBT is to facilitate and encourage teenagers to take control of their problems and to manage their lives in a healthy, progressive, less reactive and more adaptive manner.

Chapter 4

Dialectical behavioural therapy (DBT)

Dialectical behavioural therapy (DBT) was developed by Dr Marsha Linehan, a psychologist in the late 1970s at the University of Washington. This model of therapy was originally developed to treat suicidal individuals diagnosed with borderline personality disorder. DBT has proven to be extremely beneficial for those who have persistent difficulties in managing their emotions. The goal of this therapy is to teach coping skills, regulate emotions and improve relationships with others.

The DBT model of intervention focuses specifically on:

- ✓ **Distress tolerance**: Supporting teenagers in feeling and acknowledging intense emotions without reacting impulsively or negatively, in order to reduce the emotional pain they are experiencing.
- ✓ **Emotion regulation**: Accepting, labelling and regulating emotions and feelings in a positive, soothing and nurturing manner rather than in a negative, reactive manner.
- ✓ **Mindfulness**: Enhancing awareness of oneself and others while becoming attentive and aware in the here and now.
- ✓ **Interpersonal effectiveness**: Dealing with conflicts in a proactive rather than a reactive manner and interacting assertively rather than aggressively.

The components of DBT
DBT incorporates four distinct stages:

1. Attends to and deals with the most self-destructive behaviours presented, such as suicide attempts or self-injury.
2. Concentrates on quality-of-life skills, such as emotional adaptation, distress tolerance, and interpersonal efficiency.

3. Focuses on improving relationships and self-esteem.
4. Promotes life engagement and relationship connection.

The protocol for DBT treatment includes:

✓   Weekly individual therapy for approximately 50 minutes.
✓   Weekly skills training classes.
✓   Phone coaching to support and encourage teenagers to implement and utilise learned skills in crisis situations.
✓   Consultation groups that allow healthcare providers to stay motivated and discuss patient care and progress.

DBT techniques
Distract using 'ACCEPTS'
Teenagers are taught and encouraged to utilise ACCEPTS to distract themselves momentarily when feeling unpleasant emotions. 'ACCEPTS' stands for:

Activities: Engage in activities that they enjoy and derive pleasure from.

Contribute: Help and assist another person or participate in community engagement activities for the benefit of others.

Comparison: Compare themselves to people who are less fortunate and appreciate what is good in their lives. Appreciate and validate the progress they are making.

Emotions (opposite): Acknowledge their negative emotions and engage in an activity that will induce the opposite emotion – for example, if feeling sad, watch a comedy which will induce a more positive state of mind. I have found this element to be very beneficial and embraced very quickly by my teenage clients, with very positive results.

Push away: Direct the negative emotion/situation to the back of their mind; place it on the back burner to be addressed at another time – for example, when they next meet their counsellor. Let it go for now and engage in a meaningful enjoyable activity. Do not feed the Gremlin – quieten him!

Thoughts: Distract with more pleasant thoughts, memories and/or engaging activities that require concentration – for example, doing crosswords, puzzles, reading or baking. In my experience, teenagers embrace this technique very willingly and report positive results.

Sensations: Change their state of mind by engaging in a strong physical stimulus that can help to disconnect them physically from the intense pain and emotion they are currently experiencing. Examples include cold shower, hot pressure shower, and listening to loud music with a good strong uplifting beat. I tend to spend some time on this element encouraging my teenage clients to explore and try out activities that suit them specifically.

'IMPROVE' the moment
This skill is used in moments of distress to help teenagers relax and ground themselves. 'IMPROVE' stands for:

Imagery: The teenager is encouraged to imagine and visualise relaxing scenes and places he/she enjoys. Remember happy times and events and validate their progress.

Meaning: Find some purpose or meaning in what they are feeling. What lessons can be learned? What can they offer as a result of feeling this way? For example, 'I have such understanding and compassion for people who are feeling like me. I know how they feel because I have been through it.'

Prayer: Many people find peace and solace in prayer and connection to their higher being. For teenagers who are not religious and do not have a connection or belief in a higher being, meditation can be a valuable tool to utilise, focusing on inner peace and accomplishment, or connecting spirituality with oneself and nature.

Relaxation: Teenagers are taught to relax their muscles, breathe deeply and utilise self-soothing activities that work for them. Examples include listening to relaxing music, baking, engaging in exercise, having a hot bath, and cooking a nice meal to enjoy with a significant supportive person.

One thing in the moment: Focus the teenager's attention on what he/she is doing right now (helping oneself) – staying in the here and now. The aim here is to keep oneself in the present, distracted from the pain of the past, and prevent oneself from worrying about tomorrow. This is a key element in therapy and again I give due time and consideration to this technique and challenge and motivate my teenager clients to embrace it, helping them to prevent negative speculation about the future.

Vacation (brief break): This does not mean taking a holiday. Taking a vacation, in terms of the DBT model, means taking a break from the present crisis, even if only momentarily. Giving yourself a break, or a treat, by having a massage, or a facial, or a cup of tea, or taking a shower or a stroll. Engage in an activity that revives, calms and soothes.

Encouragement: Teenagers are urged to engage in positive self-talk and are encouraged to value themselves, their skills, resources and resilience. I have found encouraging teenagers to start and end the day with a positive affirmation to be extremely powerful and beneficial.

'PLEASE MASTER'

In employing this technique, DBT therapists focus on the teenager's lifestyle habits and help the teenager to realise the effects a negative lifestyle can have on physical and emotional wellbeing.

Physica**L** illness (treatment): If you are unwell or become injured, seek medical assistance immediately.

Eating (balanced): Eating crap will make you feel like crap. The importance of a healthy, balanced diet is imperative for emotional wellbeing.

Avoid mood-altering drugs: Teenagers are encouraged to avoid mood-altering substances as these substances can and will hinder emotional wellness. Only take medications under the guidance of a GP or psychiatrist and avoid alcohol.

Sleep (balanced): Sleeping too much or too little has a domino effect on physical and emotional wellbeing. Teenagers are encouraged to take the necessary steps to get their sleeping patterns back on track.

Exercise: Teenagers are encouraged to engage in regular physical activities and the benefits of doing so are clearly outlined.

Mastery: Teenagers are encouraged, challenged and motivated to do something every day that gives them a sense of competence, empowerment and achievement. I actively encourage my teenage clients to do this and record in their journal what they did and how it made a positive difference to them.

'DEARMAN'

In employing the DEARMAN technique, teenagers are taught to communicate their needs in an assertive rather than aggressive or passive manner. They are encouraged and facilitated to:

Describe factually the situation they are struggling with or having a negative reaction to.

Express why this is an issue and how they feel about it.

Assert themselves proactively by clearly asking for what they want or need.

Reinforce their position and the benefit.

Mindfully remain focused on the situation and avoid distractions.

Appear confident, even if they don't feel confident or comfortable, by maintaining eye contact, a positive open posture and an engaging tone of voice.

Negotiate and be comfortable with the outcome.

'GIVE'

Increasing GIVE skills assists teenagers in developing and maintaining positive relationships and interactions. They are taught and encouraged to develop the following key interaction skills:

Gentle: Using appropriate language, avoiding physical attacks, being courteous and non-judgemental.

Interested: Listening to others, avoiding being too opinionated and talking over people, collaborating and being patient and respectful.

Validate: Showing that they understand another person's situation and point of view by listening, paraphrasing and empathising with them.

Easy manner: Being calm and comfortable during conversation, smiling and reciprocating.

'FAST'

Teenagers are encouraged to maintain and develop their self-respect by employing and being mindful of FAST techniques:

Fair: Be fair to yourself and the people you interact with.

Apologies (few): Recognise when apologies are warranted and appropriate and offer them. Do not engage in unjustified apologies.

Stick to your values: Remain grounded and congruent. Don't allow others to manipulate or misguide you for their own benefit. Remain true to your core values which serve you well. Turn down the Gremlin's voice!

Truthful: Be honest and truthful with yourself and others.

Emotional regulation

Teenagers are taught to understand how their emotions work, develop the skills needed to manage those emotions rather than letting their emotions control them, and how to build positive emotional experiences. They learn to do so by adhering to the following steps:

- ✓ Identify and label their emotions.
- ✓ Identify obstacles to changing their emotions.
- ✓ Reduce their vulnerability to overpowering emotional states.
- ✓ Increase positive emotional states.
- ✓ Increase mindfulness to current emotions.
- ✓ Take the opposite action – for example, when a negative thought surfaces challenge it and engage in positive self-talk by giving yourself a compliment. Don't listen to the Gremlin!
- ✓ Apply 'distress tolerance techniques' – for example, do not act on distress in a negative way – that is, by self-harming – but engage in a more nurturing and soothing activity that can be enjoyed and give pleasure.

Story of emotion

This skill is used to help teenagers to understand what kind of emotion they are feeling:

- ✓ Prompting event – What is the trigger that makes you feel this way?
- ✓ Interpretation of the event – How do you view the situation?
- ✓ Body sensations – How are you feeling in your body?
- ✓ Body language – What are you communicating to others non-verbally?
- ✓ Action urge – What action do you feel like taking to reduce the distress?
- ✓ Action – What positive action can you take to manage your emotional distress?

✓   Emotion name – What exact emotion were you feeling? (Identify and understand the emotion.)

The role of the DBT therapist

The role of the DBT therapist is to:

- ✓ Ensure a non-judgemental and safe environment.
- ✓ Encourage and motivate teenagers to realise their potential and skills.
- ✓ Develop clients' skills and nurture coping mechanisms.

Research conducted by Groves *et al* (2012), and Neece *et al* (2013) found that DBT was extremely beneficial and successful for treating teenagers diagnosed with depression, as well as those who presented to mental health care professionals with suicidal thoughts, and with aggressive and impulsive behaviours.

Motivational interviewing

Motivational interviewing was developed by clinical psychologists Professor William R Miller and Professor Stephen Rollnick. Motivational interviewing is a collaborative approach that elicits behavioural changes by assisting teenagers to explore and resolve their ambivalence to change. I have found this approach to be very effective with teenagers who are less motivated. This approach aims to strengthen a teenager's motivation for and movement toward a specific goal by eliciting and exploring the teenager's own reasons for change within an atmosphere of acceptance and compassion.

Main tenet of the motivational interviewing model

The facilitator must aim to:

- ✓ Be non-judgemental
- ✓ Be non-confrontational

✓ Be non-adversarial
✓ Increase awareness of causes of problems experienced, consequences of problem behaviours, and risks faced as a result of the problem behaviours
✓ Assist teenagers to foresee a better future
✓ Motivate teenagers to achieve goals.

Role of therapist utilising motivational interviewing model

✓ The therapist must engage with and encourage the teenager to talk about their concerns, issues and hopes.
✓ The therapist must focus conversations around the behaviours and patterns that the teenager wants and needs to modify.
✓ The therapist must elicit the teenager's motivation for change by increasing the teenager's sense of the importance of change, his/her confidence about the changes required, and his/her willingness to change.
✓ The therapist in collaboration with the teenager explores and develops concrete goals and steps in order to empower the teenager to make the changes he/she desires.
✓ The therapist must always convey empathy by employing reflective listening techniques thus communicating a thorough understanding of the teenager's point of view and underlying drives.
✓ The therapist must point out and challenge any discrepancies between the teenager's values and his/her current behaviour (i.e. tease out ways in which current unhealthy behaviours conflict with his/her desires, goals and wishes).
✓ The therapist sidesteps the teenager's resistance by responding with empathy and understanding rather than confrontation.
✓ The therapist must support and develop the teenager's

self-efficacy by building his/her confidence and belief that change is possible.

✓ The therapist encourages the teenager's freedom of choice and self-direction within the parameters of safety for him/herself and others.

✓ The therapist must remain highly attentive and responsive to the teenager's motivational signs, signals and achievements.

Skills and techniques of motivational interviewing

The following skills and techniques should be used in the order in which they are listed:

1. OARS

Open-ended questions: Therapists ask questions that require more than a simple yes or no answer. Open-ended questions invite teenagers to think about and explore more possibilities and the benefits of change.

Affirmations: Affirmations are used to validate teenagers' progress towards goals and aid in confidence building and motivation.

Reflections: The therapist demonstrates to the teenager's understanding through reflective listening and empathy.

Summaries: The therapist summarises the main issues presented and any ambivalence observed. Summarising displays the therapist's understanding and capacity for actively listening to, and understanding, the teenager's frame of reference.

2. Change talk

'Change talk' is when therapists talk about change or looking forward. The therapist must be alert and attentive to teenagers' change talk, which is an indication of their commitment and motivation to change current unhealthy behaviours. The therapist must actively encourage change talk.

Examples of change talk questions I employ include:

What would you like to see change in your current situation?

Could you share with me your reasons for wanting to change this situation?

What might happen if you don't make these changes?

What could be different if you engaged and continued to come and work with me?

What would be the good things about changing your thinking and your views about your issues?

What would your life be like one year from now if you could make the changes you desire?

Why do you think … is concerned about you?

How do you think your life would be different if you could make the changes you desire?

The process used in investigating teenagers' change talk is referred to as 'DARN-CAT':

Preparatory change talk
Desire: explore the teenager's desire to change.
Ability: empower the teenager to realise change is possible.
Reason: explore the positive reasons for change.
Need: explore and define the need for change.

Implementing change talk
Commitment: uncover teenagers' commitment and motivation for change.
Activation: move teenagers from contemplation to action.
Taking steps: define goals and action steps and set targets to be achieved collaboratively.

The therapist must move the teenager from contemplating changes to implementing changes.

Research conducted by Brown *et al* (2003) found that teenagers who smoked cannabis and had a diagnosis of depression significantly decreased their cannabis use while engaged in a treatment programme utilising motivational intervention techniques.

Chapter summary – Therapeutic techniques

While each of the therapeutic models outlined has shown favourable results in lifting suicidal thinking and reducing and eliminating self-harming behaviours, we must remember that each teenager is different and unique and may take to one model more willingly and productively than another. Therapists supporting teenagers who present with suicidal ideation and self-harming behaviours need to have a sound knowledge and understanding of adolescent development and employ only therapeutic interventions in which they are adequately trained and supervised, while ensuring the modalities they advocate are based on sound scientific exploration and validation.

The ultimate goal of any therapeutic intervention is to provide teenagers with the opportunity to present and explore their problems and their reasons for self-harming and/or thinking about suicide. This involves focusing on eliciting and exploring reasons for change and for living, in order to build the motivation to change and live more productively and harmoniously. The therapist's focus must firstly be directed towards sustaining life and giving hope in the case of a teenager presenting with suicidal ideation. He/she must focus secondly on maintaining engagement in therapy, and thirdly on providing the resources, tools and the building of skills to empower teenagers to achieve the changes they require in order to live a more content, peaceful and engaging life.

Chapter 5

Complementary therapies

The whole is more than the sum of its parts.

Aristotle

The purpose of this chapter is to outline the value and function of complementary therapies and how they can be beneficial when used in association with talk therapies, medication and good diet and nutrition. Each therapy has its value, as each of us is unique – one may prefer or gain more benefit from either or of any of the outlined treatments.

Complementary treatments have grown in popularity and credibility in recent years. The treatments and interventions outlined in this chapter have proved to be beneficial in reducing stress, anxiety and regulating interrupted sleep patterns and are most beneficial when combined with talk therapies, and medication when prescribed, along with nutrition and exercise.

Holistic treatments are founded on the principle of wholeness and balancing (what the scientists call 'homeostasis'), taking into account the whole person to include the mind, body and spirit.

Holistic practitioners work on the basis that we are made up of interdependent parts; if one part is not functioning properly this will have an effect on other areas. If, for example, we are not sleeping well due to being stressed, this lack of quality sleep will hinder our quality of life. Lack of sleep can make us irritable and fatigued and more prone to angry outbursts; this in turn affects relationships and our social and emotional wellbeing. A vicious cycle begins, prompting the onset of self-defeatist syndrome.

All therapies and interventions outlined in this chapter are based on the principles of relaxation, with the ultimate goal of reducing stress and restoring balance (homeostasis) and increased energy levels.

Indian head massage

Indian head massage is based on an ancient Ayurvedic healing system which has been practised in India for thousands of years. This relaxing treatment involves massaging of the soft tissues in the upper back, shoulders, neck, arms, scalp and face. A range of different massage pressures and rhythms are employed by the therapist, aiming to invigorate these areas, unclogging tensions and blockages with a view to 'rebalancing natural energies' and 'shifting areas of negativity'. This treatment is non-invasive and very relaxing. Sessions are generally 30 to 45 minutes.

Benefits

Therapist who employ this technique do so in the hope that they may aid clients in gaining:

✓ Higher levels of alertness and concentration
✓ Relief from tension headaches
✓ Relief from insomnia
✓ Release from muscular knots and tension

✓   Improved blood circulation to the head and neck
✓   Improved lymphatic drainage from the head and neck
✓   More of a relaxed state.

Personally, I have gained great relief from tension headaches and improved my concentration and alertness after engaging in this treatment almost within hours!

Reflexology

Reflexology is a gentle healing therapy which dates back to ancient Egypt and China. In 1913 Dr William Fitzgerald introduced 'zone therapy' to the Western world. He advocated that the application of pressure to one part of the body could create a positive effect or shift in another. In the 1930s, Eunice Ingham enhanced and embraced the concept of zone therapy and defined what we now call reflexology. She is credited with uncovering and demonstrating that reflexes on the feet and hands were an exact mirror image of the organs of the body.

Reflexology is the practice of treating points and areas in the feet and hands that relate to corresponding parts of the body. A reflexologist aims to relieve stress and pain in other parts of the body through the manipulation of the feet or hands. The underlying premise of this technique is that pressure applied to certain points in the feet or hands will send signals that balance the nervous system, releasing chemicals known as endorphins, which reduce stress and pain. Employing specific hand and finger techniques, a reflexologist aims to increase circulation and induce relaxation which boosts and activates one's own healing system.

On the first visit, a reflexologist will take a full personal history, taking note of any medical conditions, lifestyle habits and reasons for seeking treatment. A reflexology treatment lasts for approximately one hour and is extremely relaxing.

Benefits

Studies which I summarise below have shown that reflexology can have the following benefits:

- ✓ Reduces anxiety levels and stress
- ✓ Induces quality sleep
- ✓ Improves circulation
- ✓ Boosts the immune system
- ✓ Increases energy levels
- ✓ Aids relaxation.

Personally I find reflexology to be very beneficial and extremely relaxing. After treatments I have found that I do in fact sleep much better. My clients have also reported sleeping better after three to four treatments.

Evidence

The scientific studies that have validated the benefits of reflexology include:

Reflexology found to reduce anxiety levels:
- Kunz and Kunz (2008) analysed 168 research studies (this is called a 'meta-analysis') published in scientific journals. Based on the studies they reviewed, they reported that reflexology created a relaxation effect. Participants who underwent reflexology were noted to have a reduction in blood pressure and a decrease in anxiety levels.

Reflexology found to relieve tension headache:
- Brendstrup and Launse (1997) conducted a study in which 78 reflexologists treated 220 patients, the majority of whom had moderate to severe headache symptoms. Three months after completing a reflexology session, 65% of patients reported that reflexology helped with

symptoms, 19% stopped taking headache medications, and 16% stated that reflexology was a cure.

- Testa (2000) conducted a blind, random trial, in which 32 patients with headaches were evaluated after several sessions of foot reflexology. Results showed that foot reflexology was as effective as drug therapy.

Therapeutic massage

Therapeutic massage dates back thousands of years. References to massage therapy appear in writings from ancient China, Rome, India, Japan, Egypt and Greece. Massage therapy is the deliberate and methodical manipulation of muscle and soft tissue with the aim of improving and supporting wellbeing within and among the various systems of the body while the body and mind are at rest.

Massage therapy incorporates several different techniques. Massage therapists will aim to manipulate muscles and other soft tissue through a process of pressing, kneading, tapping and rubbing, generally using their hands and fingers, and in some cases they may use their forearms or elbows. It is a soothing and stimulating treatment performed with the intention of influencing and boosting the body's inner energetic systems. Therapeutic massage helps to relieve associated muscular tension and brings about a state of general relaxation. Sessions generally last from 30 to 90 minutes.

Benefits

Studies which I summarise below have shown that therapeutic massage can have the following benefits:

- ✓ Releases endorphins that help to uplift the mood system and reduce depression
- ✓ Improves circulation of blood and lymph

✓ Triggers a relaxation response
✓ Invigorates the body and mind
✓ Relieves muscle tension
✓ Relieves the symptoms of tension headaches
✓ Induces quality sleep.

I personally love and derive great benefits from therapeutic massage, particularly when massage oil is infused with a few drops of aromatherapy oil, lavender being one of my favourites. During my final year in college, which was particularly demanding and stressful, I engaged in full body massage at least once a month. I found myself to be less stressed and tense in my body, particularly around my neck and shoulders.

Evidence

The scientific studies that have validated the benefits of therapeutic massage include:

Aggressive adolescents benefit from massage therapy

- Diego *et al* (2002) conducted a study in which 17 aggressive adolescents were randomly assigned to a massage therapy group to receive 20-minute therapy sessions, twice a week for five weeks. The massaged adolescents had lowered anxiety levels after the first and last sessions. By the end of the study, they also reported feeling less hostile and they were perceived by their parents as being less aggressive.

Massage reduces anxiety and depression in child and adolescent psychiatric patients

- Field *et al* (1992) conducted a study in which a 30-minute back massage was given daily over a five-day period to 52 hospitalised depressed children and adolescents. At the end of the period, the massaged children and teenagers were less depressed and anxious. In addition, nurses rated the children and teenagers as being less anxious and more cooperative, also commenting that these young people's night-time sleep had increased over the treatment period.

Aromatherapy

Aromatherapy is concerned with the psychological, physiological and pharmacological effects of essential oils through inhalation and application to the skin. It involves the use of the fragrant part of aromatic plants to improve health and general wellbeing. Appropriate fragrances can reduce stress, lift mood, increase motivation and induce quality sleep.

Evidence

The scientific studies that have supported the usefulness of aromatherapy include:

Massage combined with essential oils found to reduce anxiety and improve mood:

- Edge (2003) conducted a study in which eight participants engaged in regular massage therapy using aromatherapy oils. This study found that six of the eight participants experienced reduced anxiety and improved mood over an eight-month period.

Application

Aromatherapy oils can be used in the following ways:

- ✓ For massage, blend with a carrier oil and massage onto the body.
- ✓ While bathing, simply run a bath and add about five drops of a preferred oil (see below).

✓ For room fragrance using an oil burner. Fill the small reservoir at the top of the burner with water. The water is heated by lighting a nightlight which is placed under the reservoir. Add five drops of a preferred oil into the water. It will evaporate, filling the room with aroma. You can also rub a few drops of oil onto a cold light bulb. When the bulb is switched on and heats, the heat will cause the oil to evaporate and fill the room with its aroma.

Essential oils for relieving anxiety and depression

There is a long history of the oils listed below being credited with particular effects.

✓ **Basil** is regarded as a clearing oil and an effective aid for exam nerves, inducing the ability to concentrate and counteracting listlessness.

✓ **Bergamot** (one of my favourites) – is regarded as an uplifting oil, recommended for people who feel anxious and experience low mood.

✓ **Cedarwood** is regarded as a composing oil, recommended for people who feel stressed and who often have fleeting and scattered thoughts.

✓ **Clary sage** is regarded as a euphoric oil, recommended for premenstrual tension, insomnia, listlessness and negative thoughts.

✓ **Coriander** has been noted to stimulate appetite and is recommended for people who experience a loss of appetite.

✓ **Frankincense** is noted for its rejuvenating qualities and recommended for people who struggle with apprehension, fear, nightmares, panic attacks and self-criticism.

✓ **Geranium** is noted for its balancing qualities and has a positive effect on the lymphatic system. It is also thought to be beneficial in stabilising mood swings.

✓ **Lavender** is probably one of the most popular essential oils. It is noted for its ability to enhance the immune system, reduce stress, anxiety, negative thinking and irritability. I tend to use this quite a lot around my house and in my therapy room.

✓ **Lemongrass** is generally recognised to have strengthening properties. It is uplifting and can be beneficial for those who struggle with a lack of motivation or with exhaustion. This is another one of my favourites and I tend to burn it in my office when studying and completing assignments and paperwork.

✓ **Peppermint** is regarded for its cooling effect and widely used for nausea and migraine. It is regarded as a mental stimulant and can be beneficial for those studying for exams.

✓ **Rosemary** is noted for its stimulating qualities, both mental and physical. This oil can be effective in inducing calmness and clarity.

✓ **Ylang Ylang** is thought to aid confidence as it has a very warming aroma. It is most noted for its ability to sooth impatience, irrational thoughts and irritability.

Note!: Please seek the advice of a qualified aromatherapist if you are pregnant or considering using aromatic oils for children under 12 years of age. Essential oils should be kept away from the eyes. If you have any unpleasant reactions to any of the oils outlined, you should refrain from using it/them immediately and seek advice from a qualified aromatherapist or your local health store.

Craniosacral therapy (CST)

In the 1930s, William Sutherland (1873-1954), an osteopath, founded the field of cranial osteopathy. He detected the importance of cranial bone mobility and the consequences that restrictions in this area had throughout the whole body. CST is a delicate touch treatment that claims to enrich the body's innate capacity for healing. It is an extremely gentle therapy, which is non-intrusive and employs no levels of manipulation.

It focuses on the bones of the head, spinal column and sacrum and frees up the tissues in and around the craniosacral system to enrich the movement of cerebrospinal fluid (CSF). CSF nurtures, defends and cleanses the central nervous system and improves nerve conductivity. Enhanced flow of CSF affords the body better resources, enabling it to perform more productively, heal and restore.

CST stimulates relaxation by soothing the autonomic nervous system, which controls our 'fight or flight' response. This gentle releasing of chronic tensions within the body can effect major changes in both physical and emotional wellbeing. The goal is to release compression, which in turn alleviates stress and pain.

Benefits

Studies, including the 2012 study I have listed below, indicate that CST:
- ✓ Reduces migraines and headaches
- ✓ Reduces stress and tension-related problems
- ✓ Combats chronic fatigue.

Evidence

Scientific studies that support the use of CST include:

CST found to reduce symptoms of stress and increase levels of awareness:
- Brough *et al* (2012) reported that participants described positive changes in health-related quality of life after

engaging in CST. These changes were categorised into three domains: body, mind and spirit. Most described positive change in more than one domain. Participants reported a reduction in symptoms and altered states of consciousness and increased levels of awareness.

Several years ago I suffered a long and prolonged bout of migraines and underwent four sessions of CST over a six-week period. I found a significant reduction in symptoms after three sessions.

Acupuncture

Acupuncture originated in China and has been in use for more than 3000 years. The Western world has embraced this form of therapy and many studies validate its effectiveness. Acupuncturists work on the belief that the body's life energy, termed 'Qi', travels around the body through routes called meridians. Any illness or unease is viewed as an energy imbalance. An acupuncturist will counteract and shift these imbalances by inserting very fine needles at certain points called 'acupoints'. Needling acupuncture points stimulates the nervous system to release endorphins, which are the body's natural pain killers, into the central nervous system. This helps to reduce pain and promote healing.

During the first consultation clients are asked about their health history, lifestyle habits and reason for seeking help. The acupuncturist will also want to ascertain client goals for treatment and if the client is under the care of other health professionals. The first appointment in my experience will take approximately 60-75 minutes, whilst subsequent appointments will last approximately 45 minutes.

Benefits

Scientific evidence, including the 'meta-analysis' (study of all previous studies) listed below, indicates that acupuncture can:

✓ Stimulate the nervous system, resulting in the release of neurochemical messenger molecules. The consequential biochemical changes influence the body's homeostatic mechanisms, therefore encouraging physical and emotional wellbeing.

✓ Regulate levels of neurotransmitters and hormones, such as serotonin, noradrenaline, dopamine and GABA, which results in altering the brain's mood system, which helps to combat negative thinking, stress and anxiety

✓ Activate the parasympathetic nervous system, which induces a relaxation response.

Evidence

Research highlights that accupuncture assists in relieving the symptoms of depression:

• Mukaino *et al* (2005) conducted a meta-analysis of previous studies assessing the beneficial effects of acupuncture in cases of depression. They compiled and analysed results from 477 different research participants across eight randomised controlled trials and, based on the data collected, concluded that acupuncture was an effective treatment that could significantly reduce the severity of the experience of depression.

While I was undergoing my last IVF treatment I engaged in weekly sessions of acupuncture over a two-month period. I found myself to be more relaxed, less anxious and less tearful, with more energy during this IVF cycle than previous cycles in which I did not engage in acupuncture.

Meditation

The word 'meditate' comes from the Latin word *meditatum*, which means to ponder. Meditation is intended to promote relaxation and clear the mind, with the aim of promoting and developing self-compassion and patience. Mindful meditation develops the capacity to become more aware and to be present in the here and now. The objective is to focus and quieten the mind, promoting a higher level of awareness and inner peace.

There are many types of meditation, all involving techniques for focusing attention. The object of one's focus can be an image, an idea, a word, a phrase, or one's breathing. With continued and regular practice, meditation enables inner peace and the development of perspective. Mindfulness is a very simple and beneficial stress reduction tool.

Benefits

Evidence indicates that meditation:

- ✓ Decreases levels of anxiety
- ✓ Lowers blood pressure
- ✓ Induces a level of calmness
- ✓ Induces quality sleep
- ✓ Increases serotonin production, which improves mood
- ✓ Lowers levels of blood lactate, reducing anxiety attacks
- ✓ Sharpens the mind through gaining focus.

Evidence

Research highlights that meditation assists in reducing anxiety and symptoms associated with depression:

- A study conducted by Lee *et al* (2007) investigated the effectiveness of a meditation-based stress-management programme in patients who presented with an anxiety disorder. Forty-six patients diagnosed with anxiety disorders were randomly assigned to either a meditation programme or an education programme. The education programme focused on the biological aspects of anxiety disorders, with no stress management or behaviour techniques taught. Prescribed medications were not altered during the study. The duration of the programme was eight weeks, with one hour-long session provided weekly. There were significant decreases in all anxiety scale scores for the meditation-programme group compared with patients on the education programme.

- Goyal *et al* (2014) focused on 47 clinical trials performed in June 2013 among 3515 participants that involved meditation. Participants had sought help for various mental and physical health issues, including depression, anxiety, stress and insomnia. The study found moderate evidence of improvement in symptoms of anxiety and depression after participants underwent an eight-week training programme in mindfulness meditation.

Yoga

High stress levels result in what yoga teachers term 'vata derangement', in which one's 'air elements', associated with movement and instability, become increased. Yoga practitioners advocate that when vata levels are high and increased the person will have a 'rajasic' state of mind, being unable to focus and having constant fleeting thoughts. Typical symptoms of a vata imbalance include impatience, insomnia and anxiety.

The practice of yoga combines three elements: physical poses, controlled breathing and a short period of deep relaxation. For optimum benefits, yoga must be engaged in regularly. Yoga can help a teenager become more calm, energetic and positive.

Benefits

Evidence suggests that yoga:

- ✓ Reduces stress and tension
- ✓ Lowers blood pressure
- ✓ Reduces cortisol (stress hormone) levels
- ✓ Induces quality sleep
- ✓ Induces a feeling of connectedness with one's body and mind
- ✓ Improves concentration.

Evidence

Research has found that yoga to reduces stress and anxiety:

- Smith *et al* (2007) conducted a study in which 132 participants with mild to moderate stress levels completed a 10-week hatha yoga class of one hour per week. Results showed that the participants' stress and anxiety levels significantly reduced as a result of engaging in this 10-week yoga programme.

Chapter summary – Complementary treatments

Complementary and holistic treatments have many proven benefits, which I have experienced personally and been informed by clients of similar experiences.

Please seek the advice of a GP before embarking on any complementary treatment. Each complementary therapy has it merits, but one needs to find the one that suits the individual best in terms of what they derive most pleasure and relaxation from. One must commit to the treatment process as benefits may take time to emerge. It is important to engage with a practitioner who is fully compliant with registering bodies and is fully trained in the practice and therapy he/she is offering.

Chapter 6

Eating well for mental health

One cannot think well, love well, sleep well, if one has not dined well.

Virginia Woolf

Good nutrition is the cornerstone of positive wellbeing. Our bodies need nutrition for:

- ✓ Growth and repair
- ✓ Heat and insulation
- ✓ Energy
- ✓ Protection
- ✓ Sustained physical and emotional wellbeing.

What we eat dictates how we feel. This is known as the 'food-mood' connection. Eating CRAP will make you fell like CRAP!

C – Carbonated sugary drinks = C – Crash and crave
R – Refined sugar = R – Restless and rude
A – Artificial sweetners and colours = A – Anxious and angry
P – Processed foods = P – Panic and pain

Foods to nourish and boost your mood

In order to function well, the brain needs a balanced and ongoing supply of:

- **Complex carbohydrates** – These are made up of a chemical structure consisting of three or more sugar molecules linked together. They are rich in fibre, vitamins and minerals and take longer for your body to break down and absorb than simple sugars. This slow process helps to maintain a steady blood sugar level. Foods high in complex carbohydrates include: apples, asparagus, barley, beans, broccoli, carrots, corn, cucumbers, grapefruit, green beans, oats, onions, pears, prunes, potatoes, rice (brown) and spinach.

- **Essential fats** – The 'essential fatty acids' are the fats the human body cannot make for itself but must derive from its food. They comprise the poly-unstaturated omega-3 and omega-6 fatty acids (PUFAs). The omega-3s are an essential component of all cell membranes, ensuring our cells are sufficiently flexible and able to communicate with one another. They also contribute to improved circulation and oxygen uptake, and thereby to our levels of energy. The omega-6 poly-unsaturates are also essential, but we have more than enough of these in the modern diet (in corn and vegetable oils especially) and the important aim must be to get omega-6s and omega-3s into the right balance. It is therefore particularly important to eat foods that are rich in omega-3 fatty acids on a daily basis; their proportion in our diet has seriously declined with processed foods and the use of cheap vegetable oils. Omega-3s are derived from a fatty substance called linolenic acid that is broken down by our digestive systems to first alpha-linolenic acid (ALA), and then eicosapentaenoic acid (EPA) and docosahexaenoic acid (DHA). EPA and DHA have been shown to play a part in the prevention and treatment of depression and bipolar disorder and ALA has been shown to help in the prevention and treatment of pre-menstrual tension and high blood pressure (see page 95). Omega-3 fatty acids can be found in small quantities in beans, nuts, seeds, vegetables and whole grains, corn and sunflower but these are all much higher in omega-6 fatty acids, which we need to reduce in the modern diet as they promote inflammation without sufficient omega-3s to balance them. Fatty ('oily'), cold-water fish, such as sardines, salmon, mackerel and fresh tuna, are the richest sources of omega-3s, which are present in their EPA and DHA form and as such are more easily aborbed. Shellfish, especially scallops, also have useful amounts, as do eggs if chickens have received a diet rich in ALA. Significant plant sources of ALA include flaxseeds, chia seeds, sesame seeds (in tahini and hummus), perilla oil, purslane and walnuts. However, some people have been found to lack the enzyme needed to convert ALA to EPA and DHA and therefore must get their daily supply in the form of EPA and DHA.

- **Protein (amino acids)** – Protein forms the building blocks of our bodies and is essential for growth. It supports the development of cells and tissue integrity, aids digestion, and strengthens the immune system. Research suggests that one particular component of protein, the amino acid tryptophan, can influence positive mood. Sources of protein include: beef, black beans, cheese, cod, eggs, kidney beans, lamb, lentils, salmon, sardines, scallops, shrimp, tofu, tuna and turkey.

- **Vitamins and minerals** – These are known as 'micronutrients', which are needed by the body in only small amounts, but they are essential for physical and mental health. Vitamins and minerals boost the immune system and support growth and development. They are essential for the body's cells and organs to function and develop.

- **Water** – The human body is composed of about 60% water. It is essential for digestion, absorption, circulation, creation of saliva, transportation of nutrients, and the maintenance of our core body temperature. Not drinking enough water has implications for mental health. Mild dehydration can affect feelings and behaviour and cause irratiability, headaches and restlessness. However, you should be aware that too much water can also cause 'hyponatraemia' (that is, insufficient salts in the blood), which causes headaches and low mood and, if taken to excess, can kill; there are many reports of young people trying to re-hydrate after taking 'ecstasy' and drinking too much water, which has proven fatal in some instances.

Omega-3 fatty acids

As outlined above, omega-3 fatty acids play a vital role in brain function. They are an essential ingredient in the membranes of all cells, including nerve cells, and if replaced by other fats, such as 'trans fats', our cells cease to be able to communicate properly.

Oily fish contains significant amounts of the essential fatty acids eicosapentaenoic acid (EPA) and docosahexaenoic acid (DHA), which are essential for physical and mental health. The latest research suggests that EPA is a natural anti-depressant which aids mood stabilisation. It is thought to work by increasing blood flow throughout the body and to the brain while also having a positive impact on hormones and the immune system.

Omega-3 fats cannot be manufactured within the human body, therefore it is essential that we take them in through our diet. The best sources include salmon (wild rather than farmed), herring, mackerel, sardines, trout and fresh tuna.

Symptoms of omega-3 fatty-acid deficiency include:

✓ low energy
✓ poor recall
✓ dry skin
✓ mood swings
✓ depression.

Studies

In 2007 Hallahan *et al* at the Royal College of Surgeons in Ireland carried out research into whether omega-3 fatty acid supplementation could help 49 patients who had gone through repeated episodes of self-harming. In addition to psychiatric interventions, such as prescription drugs and limited talk therapy, the patients were also given either a placebo or a course of 1200 mg EPA plus 900 mg DHA over a three-month period. At the end of the treatment period, the group receiving omega-3 fatty acids showed considerable mental health improvements in comparison with the placebo group.

In 2010, Amminger *et al* conducted research that found that fish oil may prevent the progression of psychosis in high-risk young people aged 13-25 years. Participants who took capsules containing concentrated marine fish oil once a day for three months had significantly reduced rates of full psychosis compared with a placebo group. After 12 months it was found that these same young people had reduced negative symptoms and were more engaged with life than the placebo group.

When diet is insufficient

Teenagers who do not eat suffcient amounts of fish, which contains the essential fatty acids EPA and DHA, are well advised to take supplements. There is not yet any scientific research established in terms of the recommeded supplement dosage for those under 18 years of age. Given this, I would recommend that parents seek the advice of their GP, dietician or nutritional therapist in relation to daily dosage. The American Heart Association recommends that adults eat at least two servings of fish per week, but that should be limited to only one in teenagers because of potential contaminants in fish, especially mercury. A supplement where the oil has been distilled to remove all contaminants, including PCBs, will be indicated by having a combined EPA-DHA concentration of at least 60%.

Vitamin B

Known as the vitamin B complex, there are eight B vitamins: B1, B2, B3, B5, B6, B7, B9 and B12. These essential nutrients help convert our food into fuel, enabling us to remain energised throughout the day. All B vitamins are water-soluble, which means the body cannot store them; it is therefore vital they are ingested regularly through a healthy diet or supplements.

B1, also known as **thiamine**, helps the body make healthy new cells. B1 is often called the anti-stress vitamin because of its role in protecting the immune system. It ensures the wellness of the nervous system and plays a vital role in maintaining a positive mind set. It can help to stabilise the mood and improve memory and concentration. **B1 deficiency** can cause a decrease in alertness, and fatigue and irritability. Useful **sources** include asparagus, brown rice, cauliflower, eggs, flax, kale, liver, oatmeal, oranges, pork, potatoes, sunflower seeds, watermelon and whole grain rye.

B2, also known as **riboflavin**, works as an antioxidant to help fight 'free radicals', which are particles in the body that damage cells. B2 is also important for red blood cell production, which is vital for transporting oxygen throughout the body. B2 has been found to be an active agent in combating migraines. **B2 deficiency** can cause trembling, sluggishness, tension, migraines, stress and depression. Significant **sources** include almonds, asparagus, beef, broccoli, cheese, kidneys, leafy vegetables, liver, milk, mushrooms, prunes, salmon, tangerines, turkey and yeast.

B3, also known as **niacin**, helps to boost HDL cholesterol, which is termed 'good' cholesterol. B3 helps the body release energy from carbohydrates. This aids in the controlling of blood sugar and maintains the functions of the nervous system. **B3 defiency** can cause depression, irritability, fatigue and mood disturbances. Significant **sources** include salmon, swordfish, tuna, sunflower seeds and peanuts. Foods that contain tryptophan, which is an amino acid that the body converts into niacin, are also therefore good sources of B3; these include poultry, red meat, eggs and dairy products.

B5, also known as **pantothenic acid**, assists in breaking down fats and carbohydrates for energy. In addition, it is regarded as an anti-stress vitamin and is responsible for the production of sex and stress-related hormones, including testosterone. **Defiency** can cause low energy, restlessness, irritability, fatigue, and apathy. Significant **sources** include avocados, broccoli, cauliflower, chicken, lean pork, royal jelly, sweet potato, trout and turkey.

B6, also known as **pyridoxine**, helps the body make several neurotransmitters. Neurotransmitters are chemicals that carry signals from one nerve cell to another. Vitamin B6 is essential for normal brain development and function, and aids the body in making serotonin and norepinephrine. Some studies have indicated that vitamin B6 supplements could reduce premenstrual tension symptoms, such as moodiness, irritability, bloating and anxiety. **B6 deficiency** can cause nervousness, irritability, depression,   confusion and headaches. Significant **sources** include carrots, fish, non-citrus fruits, organ meats, peas, potatoes and spinach.

B7, also known as **biotin**, is important as it is essential for the conversion of carbohydrates into glucose, which is used to produce energy. In addition, it aids the functioning of the nervous system and psychological functioning and can be helpful in maintaining a steady blood sugar level. Its **deficency** can cause loss of appetite, fatigue, insomnia and depression. Significant **sources** include liver, kidney and other organ meats, egg yolk, soybeans, nuts and cereals.

B9, also known as **folic acid** or **folate**, is essential for good brain function and plays an important role in mental and emotional wellbeing. It is essential for the production of DNA and RNA, the body's genetic material, and is especially important when cells and tissues are growing quickly, particularly in the adolescent years. The body is unable to produce folic acid on its own so it needs to be consumed on an ongoing basis. Studies suggest that B9 may be helpful in fighting depression and preventing memory loss. **Deficiency** can result in poor recall, irritability, listlessness and sleep disturbances. Significant **sources** include asparagus, avocado, brussels sprouts, dark leafy greens, kidney beans, milk, orange juice, salmon, soybeans, spinach, turnip, wheat germ and whole grains.

B12, also known as **cobalamin**, is required in order to create red blood cells; without it megaloblastic anaemia will develop, which is characterised by extreme fatigue, muscle weakness, loss of balance, loss of appetite and weight loss, diarrhoea and nausea. B12 is also essential for keeping the nervous system healthy; without it permanent damage can develop to the peripheral nervous system. Vitamin B12 also plays a role in the creation of many of the mood-regulating brain chemicals (known as neurotransmitters), such as GABA, serotonin and dopamine. It is also needed to absorb folic acid and it helps to release energy. In addition to fatigue, weakness and peripheral neuropathy, **deficiency** can cause depression, confusion (including psychosis) and poor memory. Significant **sources** include fish, particularly shell fish, red meat, especially organ meats, poultry, eggs and dairy products, most notably cheese. (Vegans have to be very careful not to become B12 deficient and are well advised to consider taking a supplement.)

Vitamin C

Vitamin C, also known as **ascorbic acid,** is an important anti-stress nutrient. The adrenal glands, located on top of the kidneys, store the highest concentration of vitamin C within the body and monitor our 'fight or flight' response. When we are faced with a stressful situation, vitamin C is rapidly used up in the production of this stress hormone. The more stressed we are, the more cortisol is made in the body and as a result greater levels of vitamin C are required and used. Consequently, one of the biggest causes of overactive adrenal glands is stress. The adrenal glands are designed to deal with stress in small spurts rather than ongoing longer or chronic periods of stress. Chronic stress will overstretch them to the point of exhaustion and eventually they become too drained to meet the requirements of the body. Therefore it is important that teenagers who are highly stressed and anxious ensure an ongoing supply of vitamin C is consumed in their diet in order to prevent depletion.

Vitamin C is water soluble and gets used up quickly by the body; unlike all other mammals (apart from guinea pigs!) we humans cannot make it in our bodies so it is imperative we consume it in our diet. Unused vitamin C will be eliminated in our urine. The recommended daily intake of vitamin C for children aged 11-14 years is 35 mg per day. Children over the age of 15 years and adults need 40 mg per day

Vitamin C is also a powerful anti-oxidant. Oxidation reactions in the body produce 'free radicals', which chemically damage cells and contribute to the aging process. Research indicates that vitamin C can help in limiting the damaging effects of free radicals through its antioxidant activity; it has shown favour in helping to prevent or delay the development of certain cancers, cardiovascular disease, and other diseases in which oxidative stress plays a role.

Symptoms of adrenal fatigue, and consequent low cortisol levels, include fatigue, sugar or salt cravings, low blood sugar, poor sleep, depression and anxiety.

Symptoms of vitamin C deficiency include:

✓ tiredness and weakness
✓ muscle and joint pains
✓ nosebleeds
✓ slow wound healing
✓ problems fighting infections.

Significant sources of vitamin C include blueberries, broccoli, brussels sprouts, cabbage, cauliflower, cranberries, grapefruit, green and red peppers, kiwi fruit, mango, oranges, pineapple, raspberries, strawberries, spinach, tomatoes and watermelon.

Minerals

Minerals are important basic building blocks for proper nutrition and health. They are necessary for the transmission of messages through the nervous system, and for digestion and metabolism. Minerals create a healthy environment in which the body, using vitamins, proteins, carbohydrates and fats, can grow, function and aid healing.

The minerals **calcium** and **magnesium** have also been proven to be benefical in the reduction and elimination of tension. Both facilitate the relaxation of a tense and stressed nervous system. Calcium is a natural tranquiliser, while magnesium prevents anxiety, tension and nervousness.

Severe symptoms of calcium deficiency include:

✓ memory loss
✓ depression
✓ hallucinations
✓ muscle spasms
✓ numbness and tingling in the hands, feet, and face.

Good sources of calcium include cheese, fortified orange juice, fortified soymilk, kale, milk, sardines, soybeans, spinach, turnips and yogurt.

Low levels of **magnesium** can cause high blood pressure, anxiety disorders and migraines.

Good sources of magnesium include avocados, bananas, brown rice, dark chocolate, figs, mackerel, raw spinach and pumpkin seeds.

Potassium helps to oxygenate the brain, which results in clearer thinking and decision making. Stress, low blood sugar, acute anxiety and depression can result from a potassium deficiency.

Good sources of potassium include bananas, beans, dairy products, fish, kiwi fruit, lean poultry, liver, oranges, parsley, pineapples, potatoes, seeds and whole grains.

Zinc is also essential for good mental health. Zinc deficiencies have been linked to increased agitation and mood swings. The mineral can be depleted by stress and as a result levels of copper may increase. The body needs a balance of these two minerals for positive mood. Zinc is regarded as a calming neurotransmitter. The body does not store zinc so we need a daily intake of zinc to maintain adequate body levels. Symptoms of zinc defiency include hyperactivity, anxiety, irritability, nervousness and mood swings.

Good sources of zinc include avocado, beef, chicken, eggs, green beans, green leafy vegetables, mushrooms, nuts, oysters, pumpkin seeds and sesame seeds, tofu, wholegrains and lamb.

Serotonin

Serotonin is a neurotransmitter (brain chemical) that is thought to be important in the regulation of mood and sleep. Research has demonstrated that serotonin levels decline temporarily in most adolescence and this decline is thought to have a negative effect on the mood system. The brain produces serotonin from a chemical called **tryptophan**; consequently, teenagers are advised to consume the following foods which aid the stability of serotonin levels: bananas, beans, clams, cottage cheese, chicken, chick peas, dark chocolate, eggs, milk, nuts, oysters, pineapples, plums, squid, spinach and turkey.

Foods to avoid for good mental health

Refined carbohydrates: Refined carbohydrates, like sugar and white flour, have a negative effect on mood. Sugar in particular can lead to fluctuations in blood sugar levels, which have been linked to mood swings. Consuming junk food rich in refined carbohydrates, like fizzy drinks and sweets, causes blood sugar levels to spike, giving a short burst of energy followed by a drop, which leads to tiredness and irrationality.

Trans fats: These are oils that have been chemically altered through a process called hydrogenation and are present in commercially baked pastries, such as doughnuts, muffins and cakes, and in deep-fried foods, such as chips, fried chicken and chicken nuggets. Fast foods are high in trans fats and also lack omega-3 fatty acids. In our bodies they displace 'good fats', especially in our cell membranes, interfering with how our cells communicate with one another – of particular importance in the brain.

Caffeine: Caffeine is a stimulant when taken in moderate amounts and can increase mental alertness. However, when taken in higher doses it can cause anxiety, mood swings, headaches and dizziness and prevent quality sleep. More than 400 to 600 mg is excessive. Caffeine is found in coffee, tea, coke, chocolate and energy drinks like Red Bull (which is popular with teenagers).

Key nutrition tips for managing your mood

✓ Start the day with a healthy nutritional breakfast; this will supply energy to the brain and body. Whole-grain bread and cereals, milk, yogurt, eggs, and vegetable or fruit smoothy (home made) are good breakfast options.

✓ Don't skip meals. Fasting for too long can make you feel tired and irritable; aim to eat little but often – that is, at least every three to four hours.

✓ Reduce intake of foods that can negatively affect your mood, such as caffeine, alcohol, trans-fats and processed foods with high levels of preservatives, artificial flavourings and artficial colours.

✓ Reduce your intake of sugar and refined carbohydrates. These foods create a monentary high but quickly lead to a crash in mood and energy.

✓ Eat more complex carbohydrates, such as baked potatoes, whole-wheat pasta, oatmeal and whole grain breads. They will make energy release more gradual and even rather than spiking blood sugar up and down.

✓ Drink at least one and a half litres of water per day. Be mindful that mild dehydration (1-2%) can lead to headaches, irritability and loss of concentration. This level of dehydration is not enough to cause a feeling of thirst so you may not even be aware you have mild dehydration. Drink water even if not thirsty.

✓ Exercise and sunlight can reduce stress levels and promote the secretion of happy hormones.

✓ Balance your blood sugar. There is a significant link between mood and blood sugar balance. The more unbalanced your blood sugar level the more unbalanced your mood system will become.

Eating a healthy, balanced diet is a positive step towards improved mental health. Teenagers with any of the characteristics of self-defeatist syndrome need to be educated and encouraged to eat a healthy diet in order to take control of their ongoing wellbeing. Research indicates that there is a strong link between food and mood; we therefore need to encourage teenagers to improve their diet and make available to them foods that will nourish their bodies and minds and allow them to flourish.

A note about dietary supplements: Please note that, because of the potential for side effects and interactions with medications, dietary supplements should only be taken on the recommendation of knowledgeable, licensed healthcare providers. Parents are advised to seek the direction of their child's GP, dietician or nutritional therapist before buying any vitamin, mineral or other supplements for their child.

Chapter summary – Diet and nutrition

Eating a healthy, balanced diet will:

- ✓ Stimulate wellbeing by improving mood
- ✓ Increase energy levels
- ✓ Reduce stress and anxiety levels
- ✓ Boost concentration, alertness and performance
- ✓ Increase productivity and attainment
- ✓ Fight infection and disease.

Chapter 7

Parenting through 'self-defeatist syndrome'

Parenting is the opportunity for lifelong learning.

Liz Quish

Parenting a teenager in the midst of self-defeatist syndrome is a challenging and difficult task. Parental awareness, nurturing and encouragement are vital in aiding a teenager in navigating the many challenges presented by the Gremlin. In this chapter I will introduce you to the main parenting styles as identified by Diana Baumrind (a clinical and developmental psychologist) and share the views of parenting in a nurturing way as advocated by Alfred Adler, a renowned psychiatrist with a special interest in child-and-parent relationships. As many teenagers who struggle to evict the Gremlin become angry and anxious I will outline some practical tips to help you support a teenager during this challenging period in their lives.

In parenting teenagers we need to remember that all teenagers need to feel:

BONDED: They need to know they have a place where they belong, are wanted, accepted, loved and respected.

COMPETENT: They need to know they are capable, with skills, qualities and resources that they can utilise.

ENCOURAGED: They need to be stimulated, believed in, validated, supported and reassured.

Alfred Adler (1870-1937) was a philosopher and psychiatrist who proposed that we all have one basic desire and goal which is to belong and to feel loved. Adler believed that children need to feel valued, significant, and competent in order to develop a positive sense of self. He proposed that:

- ✓ Children are social beings and need to be connected to friends, family and community in order to ensure optimum mental health.
- ✓ Negative behaviour has a function and is a communication of an unmet need.
- ✓ Children need to feel secure and that they belong, and to know they are significant.
- ✓ Mistakes are opportunities for learning and moving forward.

Adler believed that parents and their style of parenting have a marked effect on children's social and emotional wellbeing. He proposed a democratic style of parenting for optimum social and emotional wellness. Democratic parenting is based on the following principles:

- ✓ Children are treated with respect, their views are given due consideration and valued.
- ✓ Rules are set by parents as they are seen as more knowledgeable. However, rules and the reasons for them are explained to children and the consequences for breaking rules are clearly outlined.
- ✓ If rules are broken, clear, consistent, logical and age-appropriate consequences are applied.
- ✓ Parents are kind but firm; discipline focuses on solutions

rather than punishment.

✓ Mistakes are seen as opportunities for learning and further development.

✓ Communication and encouragement form the cornerstone of family and individual wellness.

Research indicates that children raised in a democratic parenting style tend to be competent, and more likely to be socially and emotionally intelligent, as children parented in this fashion are valued, encouraged, listened to and respected.

Understanding parenting styles and their effects

Diana Baumrind (1927), a clinical and developmental psychologist, is highly regarded for her research on parenting styles. She proposed that parental responsiveness (how much or how little parents meet and respond to their children's needs) and parental demandingness (the level of behavioural control parents exercise on their children based on their expectations of appropriate and acceptable behaviour) had a significant impact on children's wellbeing. Through her extensive research with children and parents she formulated the following three parenting styles.

The permissive parenting style

Permissive parenting, also known as indulgent parenting, is a model of parenting which is responsive rather than demanding. Parents who raise their children using this model generally avoid confrontations, make few demands and communicate few expectations of their children, and rarely discipline them while affording them a lot of freedom. Such parents are more concerned with being their children's friend than setting limits, rules and boundaries. This model of parenting is more child-adult led than adult-child led.

Characteristics of permissive parenting

- ✓ Parents set a limited number of rules and standards of acceptable behaviour.
- ✓ When rules are set they are more often than not inconsistent and inconsistently enforced.
- ✓ Parents behave more like friends than parents.
- ✓ They are usually very nurturing and loving towards their children.
- ✓ They tend to use enticements, such as toys, gifts and food, as a means to get their children to do as they require at certain times.

The effects of permissive parenting

Children of permissive parents are more likely than others to:

- have inadequate social skills as this parenting style is completely child focused; concern for others' feelings and experiences may not be fully realised;
- become rebellious and defiant when their wishes are not granted. Children who are raised through this model tend to have their wishes granted by parents and therefore may find it difficult to accept that they cannot have their own way all the time as they develop and navigate the wider social world;
- appear apprehensive due to a lack of boundaries and guidance from their parents.
- On a positive note, children parented in this way tend to be creative, self-confident and playful.

Lamborn *et al* (1991) conducted a study to ascertain the effects of parenting employing a permissive style. After surveying over

4000 American families who parented using this model their research concluded that teenagers parented in a permissive fashion underachieved academically and were more likely to engage in self-destructive activities such as drinking and experimenting with drugs.

Authoritarian parenting style

Authoritarian parenting is a model that is overtly strict, directive, non-collaborative, conditional, and lacks warmth and encouragement. Authoritarian parents have very high expectations of their children and set very strict rules that they expect to be followed without question. Parents who utilise this model to parent their children engage in punishments rather than discipline. Children raised by authoritarian parents are not encouraged or facilitated to explore or act independently.

Characteristics of authoritarian parenting
Authoritarian parents:

- ✓ have strict rules and expectations;
- ✓ are demanding and non-receptive;
- ✓ lack warmth and do not communciate openly;
- ✓ apply punishments with little or no explanation;
- ✓ do not offer children choices or options.

The effects of authoritarian parenting
Children of authoritarian parents are more likely than others to:

- ✓ act more aggressively outside the home environment;
- ✓ be fearful or overly shy around others;
- ✓ have diminished self-esteem;
- ✓ find difficulty forming or offering opinions;
- ✓ be very angry, resentful and frustrated;

✓   develop a fear of failure due to parental high expectations
     and the anticipated consequences of not meeting these
     expectations.
✓   However, children parented in this manner tend to
     be obedient and respectful towards their elders and
     authority figures.

Research conducted by Wolfradt *et al* (2003) found that
teenagers parented in an authoritarian fashion were more likely
to experience bouts of anxiety in situations that are unfamiliar
and demanding.

Authoritative parenting style

Authoritative parents discipline rather than punish their children.
They discipline in an age-appropriate, logical and consistent
manner. Authoritative parents are also flexible, attentive and
nurturing, displaying a balance of firmness and fairness. They
encourage their children to be independent while maintaining
age-appropriate limits and boundaries. They encourage open
communication, exploration and discussion.

Characteristics of authoritative parenting
Authoritative parents:

✓   listen to and engage with their children;
✓   encourage and promote age-appropriate levels of
     independence;
✓   set consistent age-appropriate limits, consequences and
     expectations;
✓   express warmth and openness;
✓   encourage children to express and discuss options and
     negotiate.

The effects of authoritative parenting style

Children of authoritative parents are more likely than others to:

- ✓ be more confident;
- ✓ have developed good emotional understanding and empathy;
- ✓ demonstrate good communication skills;
- ✓ be interactive and responsive;
- ✓ have a well-developed sense of self and good self-esteem;
- ✓ be willing to challenge themselves.

Research by Liem *et al* (2010) found that children parented in an authoritative fashion displayed fewer symptoms of depression during young adulthood, concluding that authoritative parenting promotes psychological wellbeing beyond childhood.

Parenting styles and you

The parenting styles outlined can best be understood as archetypical in that they are presented as clean-cut personalities and behaviour patterns. However, the majority of people don't fit neatly into one archetype all the time; rather, people behave according to one primary archetype in most situations but often fluctuate between different parenting styles during different circumstances. In supporting a teenager in the midst of self-defeatist syndrome, parents are advised to utilise a democratic and authoritative approach as these approaches have been found to be beneficial in supporting social and emotional wellness.

Parenting the angry teenager

Anger is a secondary emotion in response to an unmet need and requires a trigger. It is not always appropriate, but there are times when it *is* appropriate; this rests on how it is communicated and managed. Dr Timothy Murphy, author of *The Angry Child: Regaining Control When Your Child Is Out of Control*, proposed the following reasons for, and stages of, anger.

Three primary emotions behind anger

In supporting a teenager who is angry it is important to have an understanding of why the teenager has become angry in the first instance. Once the reason for their anger has been uncovered, then you can move to the next stage and help the teenager to manage and express their anger appropriately. Before you intervene, be aware that the teenager may be feeling;

1. Hurt: as a result of feeling rejected or feeling a sense of injustice.
2. Fearful: as a result of feeling unsafe, insecure, uncertain or having no control.
3. Frustration: as a result of being treated unfairly, failing or losing.

The stages of anger

In seeking to help teenagers who are angry it is useful to be aware of how anger develops. Dr Murphy proposes the following stages of anger.

Stage One: Lead-up, caused by:

- ✓ Past negative experiences and reactions
- ✓ Learned and observed behaviours
- ✓ Physical and emotional stress
- ✓ Poor coping skills and emotional soothing.

Stage Two: The trigger, caused by:

- ✓ Sight, sound or thought of something unpleasant
- ✓ 'Hot button' words or topics (see page 114)
- ✓ Unpleasant experiences, accidents, unplanned events or circumstances
- ✓ Immature and illogical emotional brain reasoning.

Stage Three: The outburst, which results in:

- ✓ Verbal aggression towards others
- ✓ Physical aggression towards other
- ✓ Self-harming behaviours.

Stage Four: The Aftermath

This fourth stage is very important and is often overlooked. The Aftermath is where you and the teenager need to calmly discuss and confront the original problem. Remember, whatever is unresolved is likely to become the lead-up and trigger for the next angry explosion.

Resolve the problem and gain insight to pre-empt and hopefully avert future episodes. To do this productively you need to be mindful of these principles:

- ✓ Do not threaten or respond with anger.
- ✓ Talk over what happened when you are both calm and collected; remember that the teenager's anger may not be directed at you but rather towards you – that is, the teenager may be angry and upset about an event that you are not aware of; feeling overwhelmed by the event, they may take their upset and dissatisfaction out on you.
- ✓ Look beyond the explosion for the true trigger and problem solve.
- ✓ Manage any micro-outbursts, actively listen and

summarise so the teenager knows you have heard him/ her and understand.

✓ Assist the teenager to identify and label the true emotion and develop new awareness.

Common 'hot buttons' and triggers for teenagers

Though it may seem obvious that these can spark trouble, it is very important to bear in mind at all times that the following are likely to lead to outbursts:

✓ Being lectured and nagged.

✓ Generalised negative labelling: 'You are always the same'; 'You are so lazy'; 'You can't do anything right'.

✓ Ongoing negative future predicting: 'You won't pass your exams'; 'You won't get into college'; 'You will never amount to anything', 'You will never hold down a job'.

✓ Instant problem solving: giving instant solutions rather than engaging in a collaborative discussion; talking when the teenager needs you to just listen.

Key tips for helping the angry teenager

The teenager who struggles with anger can often appear hostile and demanding. However, parents must remember that their teenager is reacting instinctively to an unmet need and must be handled with care and compassion. The following are more generalised strategies that parents can utilise to calm and support their angry teenager.

✓ Confront one problem at a time, taking a collaborative, solution-focused stance.

✓ Attend to and focus on what is reasonable and realistic for the teenager at the present time.

✓ Set ground rules with firmness and fairness, being clear and consistent about what is negotiable and what is not.

Parenting the anxious teenager

We all experience anxiety from time to time, having a few butterflies in our tummy before an exam or job interview, for example. This level of anxiety is normal and healthy and can motivate us to perform at our optimum level. However, when we become anxious and perceive a threat to our wellbeing, we activate our 'fight-or-flight' response in order to protect ourselves.

When our fight-or-flight response is activated we react to a threat in the following ways:

✓ Psychologically – we have negative thoughts.
✓ Physiologically – we experience tension in our body.
✓ Behaviourally – we take actions to sooth ourselves and seek reassurance, which can be negative or positive.

The **psychological reaction** manifests itself as:

✓ Fear – 'I am in danger...'
✓ Panic – 'I can't deal with this...'
✓ Irrational thoughts
✓ Negative thoughts
✓ Rushing thoughts
✓ Forgetfulness and disorganisation.

The **physiological reaction** manifests itself as:

✓ Heart rate increase
✓ Shortness of breath
✓ Nausea

✓ Feeling clammy and sweaty
✓ Trembling
✓ Tingling
✓ Chest pain
✓ Headache.

The **behavioural reaction** manifests itself as:

✓ Inappropriately laughing and giggling (nervous laughing)
✓ Crying
✓ Avoiding
✓ Pacing about
✓ Fidgeting
✓ Self-harming
✓ Talking very fast and incoherently
✓ Over-checking; ritualised actions
✓ Nail biting
✓ Chain smoking.

Key tips for helping the anxious teenager

The teenager who struggles with anxiety can often appear unreasonable, difficult, overly sensitive, inflexible and taxing. However, parents must remember that their teenager is reacting instinctively to a perceived threat and must be handled with care and compassion. There are many different types and levels of anxiety problem, which require specialised intervention and strategies. The following are more generalised strategies that parents can utilise to support and comfort their anxious teenager.

✓ Be patient and appreciate your teenager's anxiety is a result of a perceived threat to his/her wellbeing.
✓ Connect with your teenager and demonstrate empathic

listening, allowing him/her to voice his/her feelings and concerns; this is vital, as internalising them could lead to episodes of self-harming.

✓ Help your teenager to challenge automatic negative thoughts and the reality of these thoughts.

✓ Educate yourself and your teenager about anxiety, its triggers and manifestations.

✓ Encourage your teenager to work through his/her fears in a proactive rather than reactive manner. Do not rush him/her; let him/her work at his/her own pace. Professional help may be required depending on severity.

✓ Resist giving reassurances unnecessarily, but do encourage your teenager to utilise the nurturing coping skills that he/she will have learned if engaged with a professional.

✓ If your teenager is seeking support from a professional, become involved and seek his/her advice on how to manage your child's anxiety. Be aware of the tools and tips he/she is teaching your child and reinforce these at appropriate times.

✓ Recognise progress and validate it by reminding the teenager that he/she can gain control.

✓ Don't over-react to the teenager's anxiety as this can raise his/her stress levels. Engage in finding collaborative solutions.

✓ Encourage your teenager to establish a routine for eating, sleeping, engagement with family and friends, studying and relaxation.

✓ Work in partnership: involve and educate all family members on how to help the teenager manage and cope with a bout of anxiety if it manifests while in his/her company.

✓ Do not become passive or over-compensating. Help the teenager deal with his/her anxiety by being empathic and understanding rather than taking a passive stance. Encourage independence and involvement. Anxious teenagers will generally try to avoid things that cause them anxiety. Try not to facilitate your teenager to avoid situations and events as this could lead to isolation. Instead, encourage him/her to try and take small steps towards facing his/her fears.

✓ If your teenager becomes overwhelmed by a task, help him/her to break the task down into small steps: 'Firstly we will…, and when that is done then we can… and when that step is achieved then we can… How does that sound?' 'Let's give it a go and see.' Encourage and praise each step achieved.

✓ REPEAT!

Chapter summary – Parenting teenagers who struggle with their feelings and emotions

As I said at the beginning of this chapter, parenting a teenager in the midst of self-defeatist syndrome is a challenging and difficult task. Parental awareness, nurturing and encouragement are vital in aiding a teenager in navigating the many challenges presented by it. Depression, suicidal thoughts, self-harming, anxiety and angry outbursts can be managed and overcome once the reasons for the behaviours have been identified and dealt with in a timely fashion. Following the recommendations outlined in previous chapters will assist teenagers to evict the uninvited Gremlin.

Chapter 8

Bereavement through suicide

What we have once enjoyed deeply we can never lose. All that we love deeply becomes a part of us.

Helen Keller

Losing a child through suicide is a devastating experience. Life's course for those left behind is forever altered. Hopes and dreams are shattered, life's meaning is questioned, the pain is unbearable, and the realisation is too much to comprehend. Grieving the loss of a child through suicide is a very complex, personal and lifelong process. In this chapter, by outlining the theories of grief, I aim to give you a better understanding of the grief process which I hope will be beneficial to you if you have lost your child through suicide. I will also highlight key tips for those of you who may be supporting parents who have lost their child through suicide.

Understanding the terminology

Let me first introduce you to the common terms used by professionals in relation to a loss through death:

Grief: is the process of reacting to a loss.

Bereavement: is the process of living with and experiencing loss.

Mourning: is the outward expression of one's loss.

Theories of grief

To help those trying to cope with grief and loss, psychologists, psychiatrists and researchers have tried to understand it by analysing its constituents and stages. This insight can be helpful to those who are bereaved and to those who endeavour to support them.

Kübler-Ross's five stages of grief (1969)

Elizabeth Kübler-Ross, MD (1926–2004) was a Swiss-born psychiatrist, and the author of a very popular and well-regarded book called *On Death and Dying* (1969), in which she proposed what is now known as the Kübler-Ross model. In this work she proposed the following Five Stages of Grief as a pattern of adjustment

1. **Denial**: On hearing of the death of their cherished child through the tragedy of suicide, parents react with denial, which is a very normal and expected response. Denial is a defence mechanism that is utilised in order to shut out the reality and magnitude of a particularly stressful situation.

2. **Anger**: Once the reality of the situation penetrates a parent's emotional core, intense feelings of anger emerge. Anger can be directed towards their child for completing suicide and leaving them. It can also be directed inwards, in which case parents become very angry with themselves and each other, feeling they in some way let their child down. Anger can also be misplaced and directed towards others, as the reality of their loss becomes real and denial has lifted.

3. **Bargaining**: In the case where parents have lost their child through suicide, bargaining emerges as feelings of guilt develop. 'If only I had known what he was thinking'; 'If only I had known how much pain she was in'; 'If only I had asked'. Bargaining manifests as a result of a deep yearning for the painful and distressing situation to be reversed. During this stage, parents focus on the past so they can be spared momentarily from experiencing the pain of the reality of their tragic loss.

4. **Depression**: As the reality of losing their precious child unfolds, parents enter a state of depression as intense feelings of emptiness, abandonment, yearning, loss, isolation and sadness emerge. Life will never be the same again. Feelings of uncertainty and fear materialise as they confront and negotiate the painful reality of their huge loss.

5. **Acceptance**: When parents experience such a significant trauma as losing a child through suicide, acceptance seems like an unattainable task. Kübler-Ross seems to respectfully propose that parents may never accept the loss of their child through suicide but can and do learn to re-negotiate life and live with the reality of their loss.

Worden's four tasks of mourning (1991)

Dr William Worden, author of *Grief Counselling and Grief Therapy*, is one of the founding members of the Association of Death Education and Counselling and a pioneer in the hospice movement in the US. Worden proposed the following four tasks of mourning:

1. **Acknowledge the loss**: Parents who have lost their child through suicide will initially respond with disbelief and denial. This is a very normal grief response given the enormity of such a significant and tragic loss. Worden proposes that parents must come to the realisation that

their child has died on a cognitive (intellectual) and emotional level; once parents eventually overcome the denial stage they will then be enabled to move onto the next task of grieving, which is to feel the enormity of their very significant loss.

2. **Feel the pain**: Grief is a very painful experience. All that was familiar, loved, appreciated and nurtured is no longer physically present. This realisation causes so much pain and anguish. Worden advocates that parents must express and feel these extremely painful sensations and not try to avoid them as doing so will prevent them from achieving the next task of grieving, which, according to Worden, is to adjust to life without their precious loved child.

3. **Adjust to the new environment**: Living life without one's child after their death by suicide can seem like an insurmountable task. Many parents can feel disloyal to their child as they move on with life, albeit a very different life. Worden advocates that parents need to re-evaluate their life as it now presents without their much loved and cherished child and adjust their roles, expectations, hopes and dreams if they are to be enabled to live with the reality of their loss.

4. **Re-invest in learning to live again**: Learning to live again, albeit in a very different way, is the final task of grieving as set forth by Worden. When parents can connect with the memory of their deceased child with love, empathy, and self-compassion then they will be enabled to live again and experience positive connections and re-engage with life more fully.

Rando's six 'R' process of mourning (1993)

Researcher and clinical psychologist Therese Rando has also contributed a stage model of the grief process that she observed people to experience while adjusting to a significant loss. She called her model the 'Six R's':

1. **Recognising the loss**: This is similar to Worden's first task of acknowledging the loss. Parents must comprehend and acknowledge on a cognitive level that their child has died.

2. **Reacting to the separation**: This stage, as proposed by Rando, is comparable with Worden's second task. Parents must move from denial, and experience and express their deeply felt pain, anguish and sorrow.

3. **Recollect and re-experience** the relationship through reviewing and remembering: Parents need to, and must be encouraged to, talk about and remember significant events, achievements, challenges, talents and character traits associated with their child.

4. **Relinquish**: Parents who are navigating and moving through this stage will begin to realise on a cognitive level that life will now be different; things cannot and will never be the same now that their child had died.

5. **Readjust**: Parents begin the process of returning to daily life, tasks and chores.

6. **Reinvent**: Parents begin to form and develop new relationships, make new commitments and begin to live with the reality of their loss.

Stroebe and Schut's dual process model of bereavement (1999)

Margaret S. Stroebe, PhD, is associate professor of psychology at Utrecht University in the Netherlands. She is co-author (with Wolfgang Stroebe) of *Bereavement and Health* (1987) and (with Robert O. Hansson) of *Bereavement in Late Life* (2007) and an editor of the *Handbook of Bereavement Research: Consequences, Coping, and Care* (2001).

Henk Schut, PhD, is also associate professor of psychology at Utrecht University. His research interests cover processes of coping with loss and the efficacy of bereavement care and grief therapy. He is one of the authors of the Dutch publication *Suicide and Grief* (1983), co-author of *Individual Grief Counselling*, and one of the editors of the *Handbook of Bereavement Research: Consequences, Coping, and Care* (2001).

Together, Stroebe and Schut (1999) developed a dual process model of bereavement, advocating two tasks associated with it:

1. **Loss-oriented activities and stressors**: Parents will express and experience an array of frightening and unfamiliar feelings on the death of their child. These include crying, hankering, and feeling a great sense of sadness, denial and anger, while also staying stuck in the past and dwelling on the circumstances of their loss, and avoiding restoration activities.

2. **Restoration-oriented activities and stressors**: These include adjusting to life without their child and negotiating a new role, dealing with the many changes presented as a result of such a substantial loss, developing new ways of connecting with family and friends, and navigating a new way of life.

Stroebe and Schut suggested that parents will invariably fluctuate between the two processes.

How do these models of grief help us?

While the models of grief and bereavement I have outlined give us a greater understanding of the grieving process, we need to be mindful that grief reactions for each individual are very personal and unique. There is not a correct way to grieve, and no set pattern to follow; rather, there are common experiences, reactions and processes that each parent may experience as he/she moves through his/her grief. Exactly what these experiences and reactions will be are determined by many factors, such as one's personality type, age and health status, spiritual and religious beliefs, cultural identity, previous losses, supports and resources, and the nature of the relationship with their deceased child. Parents grieving the loss of their child in such tragic circumstances will fluctuate between the different stages, or 'tasks', of grief and mourning. As they journey through their grief and the many challenges of renegotiating a life without their precious child, most will begin to engage with life again, albeit a very different life, as they begin living with the reality of their significant loss. For some, their grief may become all too consuming, and in such circumstances they may experience what is termed 'complicated grief'.

Complicated grief

Complicated grief is a chronic, intense state of ongoing, long-lasting and debilitating grief that takes over the grieving person's life. Parents who experience complicated grief find it extremely difficult to function and engage with life on any level. They will journey back and forth through the stages and tasks of grief outlined without any concrete resolution. Shear *et al* (2005) conducted a randomised control trial (that is, a scientific trial in which the participants are randomly assigned to different treatments and do not know which they are receiving) on the treatment of complicated grief and found that 10-20% of bereaved participants experienced complicated grief reactions.

Worden (2005) outlines four categories of complicated grief reactions:

1. **Chronic grief:** This looks like typical grief reactions but the 'symptoms' do not diminish but rather persist and

may increase over a prolonged period of time.

2. **Delayed grief**: This describes typical grief reactions that are suppressed or postponed in a conscious effort not to deal with the pain of one's loss.

3. **Exaggerated grief**: This is indicated by negative and destructive coping mechanisms, such as an increase in smoking and drinking, self-medicating and overworking.

4. **Masked grief**: This is characterised by a lack of awareness and appreciation that the behaviours that interfere with normal functioning are a result of one's loss.

Signs and symptoms of complicated grief

Complicated grief is recognised as a diagnosable condition which affects up to 10% of bereaved people. Parents who lose their child through the tragedy of suicide may be more susceptible to complicated grief given the enormity of such a loss. Features that may indicate grief has become complicated grief include:

✓ Having an extended and total focus on one's significant loss

✓ Extreme and penetrating longing and yearning for one's loved one

✓ Inability to accept one's loss on a cognitive and emotional level

✓ Continued incapacitating distress and sorrowfulness

✓ Increase in self-defeating activities such as excessive drinking, over-medicating with prescription drugs and drug use

✓ Ongoing detachment

✓ Marked hopelessness and the incapacity to re-engage with life

✓ Difficulty carrying out normal daily routines, tasks and chores

✓ Retreating and isolating oneself from family, friends and
  social activities
✓ Finding life and living unbearable
✓ Ongoing irritability, anxiety and tension
✓ Obsessive ruminating and self-blame
✓ Long-lasting bouts of depression.

Grieving the loss of a child through suicide is a complicated process. However, for parents who experience ongoing, debilitating and lasting complicated grief reactions generally beyond six to 12 months, professional support and intervention are warranted and strongly advised.

Bereavement counselling

Bereavement counsellors will empathically and compassionately facilitate and support bereaved parents in realising the reality of their loss during the early stages of therapy. Parents must first accept the reality of their loss on a cognitive (intellectual) level before they can be enabled to experience and express the emotional impact of their significant loss. Through empathy, patience and understanding, a counsellor will encourage bereaved parents to talk about their child and the impact of the loss, share and express feelings, and adjust to living with the reality of their loss.

In some cases, parents may intentionally supress their feelings because of the overwhelming pain it can trigger. This needs to be addressed, as avoiding and suppressing feelings has been found to manifest in psychosomatic symptoms for some people, and ongoing psychological distress. Feelings such as guilt, anxiety, anger, hopelessness, helplessness, abandonment and loneliness can be difficult and frightening feelings to acknowledge and express. A bereavement counsellor will assist parents in normalising their feelings in a safe manner, supporting and encouraging them to name, identify and explore their feelings in order to resolve, manage and overcome them.

A bereavement counsellor will also encourage parents to share and discuss the problems they have been experiencing since the death of their child and identify coping skills, paying particular attention to any maladaptive coping mechanisms that may develop. Maladaptive coping skills include avoiding friends and family, excessive drinking, drug abuse and supressing difficult emotions. These need to be uncovered and explored with the ultimate aim of helping the parents to develop more nurturing and productive coping skills as they navigate and redefine a life without their child.

The S.U.I.C.I.D.E of suicide

I have found the following to be a useful way to summarise the challenge of helping parents who have lost a child through suicide:

S Sudden: The sudden death of a child through suicide is a life-altering experience. One does not get over the loss, but in time parents can learn to live with the reality of this very significant and traumatic loss.

U Unbelievable: A great sense of shock and disbelief emerges instantly and will continue and fluctuate for some time. The enormity of a child's tragic loss through suicide will initially be met with feelings of denial and ultimate dismay. These feeling are normal and to be expected given the magnitude of such a loss.

I Intentional: Realising that their child has died in such a traumatic, intentional and lonely manner will set parents on a life-changing and complicated journey.

C Complicated: Thoughts about not being able to cope and go on are normal grief reactions given the significance of losing a child through suicide. Parents may also think about their own suicide as a means to escape the anguish and turmoil felt as a result of losing their child in such a harrowing manner.

I   Isolating: Parents can experience a great sense of isolation, rejection and abandonment. They may feel rejected and abandoned by their child and may isolate themselves from family and friends as they try to navigate a range of unfamiliar and frightening feelings.

D   Demobilising: Depressive episodes can present on an ongoing basis as parents struggle to comprehend the enormity of their loss.

E   Engagement: Engagement with life can seem like an impossible and overwhelming task for parents who have lost their child through suicide. Life cannot and will not ever be the same. However, parents can and do re-engage with life. This is after a long and challenging journey of renegotiation and redefinement.

Supporting grieving parents

If this loss is not your own, but has happened to family or friends who need your support, here are some pointers to remember:

✓   Listen with compassion and acknowledge the tragedy and significance of losing their child through suicide.

✓   Accept and acknowledge the feelings displayed. Let the person you are supporting know it's okay to cry and feel angry and hopeless given the trauma they have experienced.

✓   Sit with the silence. Don't press the person you are supporting to talk and open up. Your presence may be all they need.

✓   Don't ask too many questions or details about their

child's death; let parents give you as much or as little information as they feel comfortable with.

✓ Allow and facilitate the person you are supporting to talk, talk and talk. Be patient. Retelling their story is a means of processing their loss.

✓ Be aware that bereaved parents are dealing with and negotiating a very significant loss and may not reach out for your help. Take the initiative and check in regularly.

✓ If you feel unsure about what to say, be honest, and share this.

✓ Share the positive things you remember about their child and what their child meant to you if you had a relationship with their child.

✓ Be aware of the terminology you use; avoid using statements like 'committed suicide' as this implies the committal of a crime. The act of suicide was decriminalised in the Irish state in 1993, in Northern Ireland in 1966 and in England and Wales in 1961. (Suicide was never an offence under Scots law.)

✓ Offer practical assistance, such as helping with shopping, dropping and collecting their other children to/from school and extra-curricular activities and helping with housework etc.

✓ Offer additional support on significant days, such as their child's birthday and the anniversary of his/her death. Be particularly mindful of parents' reactions and vulnerabilities when their child's friends reach and celebrate significant milestones – for example, exam results, graduations, engagements and weddings. Their experience of hopelessness and the significance of their loss may become heightened during these times.

✓ Remember your support may be more crucial and valuable once the funeral is over, as parents begin to journey and negotiate the many challenges of living with the painful reality of living without their child.

✓   Look after yourself and build your own support network.

Avoid using statements like:

- 'I know how you feel.' No matter what our experiences are, we cannot truly know how another person feels. Ask the person you are supporting how he/she feels so you may gain an understanding of his/her true feelings and respond empathically.
- 'Look at what you have to be thankful for.' Parents grieving the loss of their child through suicide will not be in an emotional or cognitive state to appreciate anything in life for some time.
- 'You should' or 'You will'. Instead use 'Have you thought about...' or 'You might consider...'

Chapter summary – Bereavement through suicide

Grieving for the loss of a child through suicide is clearly a complex phenomenon which presents parents with many psychological challenges as they try to negotiate a life without their child. Losing a child to suicide is difficult to comprehend and to accept such a loss disrupts the normative laws of nature and orderliness of life. The fact that a cherished and much-loved child's death entailed an element of choice raises many painful and unanswered questions; this, coupled with a range of intense, frightening and unfamiliar feelings, makes a bereavement through suicide a unique and very personal experience which is inevitably life altering. No one ever gets over the loss of their child through suicide, but rather, with the passage of time, the development of self-compassion and the ongoing support of others, parents come to live with the reality of such a significant and traumatic loss.

Appendix

Where to get help and support

Ireland

3Ts

'Turning the Tide of Suicide': 3Ts is a registered charity in Ireland, founded in 2003 to raise awareness of the issue of suicide and to raise funds to help prevent future deaths by suicide through dedicated research, intervention and support.
3 Arkle Road, Sandyford,
Dublin 18
Tel: 01 2139905
 Email: 3ts@alburn.com
Website: www.3ts.ie

Aware

Aware provides information, education and support to those affected by depression. Aware currently provides an education programme to secondary school students called Beat the Blues as well as a life skills programme that trains people how to manage mild to moderate depression and anxiety.
Aware National Office, 72 Lower Leeson Street,
Dublin 2
Tel: 01 661 7211
Email:info@aware.ir
Website: www.aware.ie

Console

A national organisation supporting people in suicidal crisis and those bereaved by suicide through professional counselling, support and helpline services. Console is a national service with centres in Dublin, Cork, Galway, Limerick, Kerry, Athlone, Wexford, Mayo and Kildare. Console is also located in London, United Kingdom.
Console House, 4 Whitethorn Grove,
Celbridge, Co Kildare
Tel: 01 610 2638
Email: info@console.ie
Website: www.console.ie

GROW

GROW is a mental health organisation which helps people who have suffered, or are suffering, from mental health problems. Members are helped to recover from all forms of emotional distress, or indeed, to prevent such happening. GROW has a range of outreach services across Ireland and Northern Ireland.
Barrack Street, Kilkenny,
Co Kilkenny
Tel: 056 61624
Email: info@grow.ie
Website: www.grow.ie

Headstrong

Headstrong is the National Centre for Youth Mental Health. Headstrong works with communities and statutory services to empower young people to develop the skills, self-confidence and resilience to cope with mental health challenges.
16 Westland Square, Pearse Street,
Dublin 2
Tel: 01 4727 010
Email: info@headstrong.ie
Website: www.headstrong.ie

Appendix

HeadsUp

HeadsUp is a youth mental health promotion project run by the Rehab Group. It provides a number of initiatives including ASIST and SafeTalk training, Lifeskills courses, text service and CBT-based online skills courses.

Roslyn Park, Sandymount,
Dublin 4
Tel: 01 2057200
Email: info@headsup.ie
Website: www.headsup.ie

Mental Health Ireland

MHI is a national voluntary organisation with 104 local Mental Health Associations and branches throughout the country. The membership includes mental health professionals and lay people who provide care, support and friendship for the mentally ill. Mental Health Ireland aims to promote positive mental health and to actively support persons with a mental illness, their families and carers by identifying their needs and advocating their rights.

Mensana House, 2 Marine Terrace,
Dun Laoghaire, Co Dublin
Tel: 01 284 1166
E-mail: info@mentalhealthireland.ie
Website: www.mentalhealthireland.ie

Pieta House

Pieta House provides a free, therapeutic approach to people who are in suicidal distress and those who engage in self-harm. Pieta House is a national service with centres in Kerry, Lucan, Limerick, Roscrea, Tallaght, Tuam, Ballyfermot, Cork and Finglas.

6 Main Street Upper,
Lucan, Co Dublin

Tel: 01 6282111
Email: mary@pieta.ie
www.pieta.ie

Reach Out

ReachOut.com is a web-based Irish service that supports
teenagers. Its aim is to improve young people's mental health
and wellbeing by building skills and providing information,
support and referrals.
Inspire Ireland Foundation,
1st floor, 29-31 South William Street,
Dublin 2
Tel: 01 764 5666
Email: info@inspireireland.ie
Website: http://ie.reachout.com/

Samaritans

Samaritans is a confidential emotional support service for
anyone in the UK and Ireland. The service is available 24 hours
a day for people who are experiencing feelings of distress or
despair, including those which may lead to suicide. Samaritans
provide services in Ireland, England, Scotland and Wales.
Tel: (for Ireland) 01 6710071
Email: jo@samaritans.org
Website: www.samaritans.org

Shine

'Supporting People Affected by Mental Ill Health': Shine is
the national organisation dedicated to upholding the rights
and addressing the needs of all those affected by enduring
mental illness including, but not exclusively, schizophrenia,
schizo-affective disorder and bi-polar disorder. Shine runs a
confidential helpline and has offices in Dublin, Cork, Galway,
Kilkenny, Tullamore and Dundalk.

38 Blessington Street,
Dublin 7
Tel: 1890 621631
Email: phil@shineonline.ie
Website: www.shineonline.ie

SOS – Suicide or Survive
SOS is an Irish charity focused on breaking down the stigma
associated with mental health issues and ensuring that those
affected have access to quality recovery services that are right
for the individual.
Stonebridge House, Stonebridge Close,
Shankill, Co Dublin
Tel: 1890 577 577
Email: info@suicideorsurvive.ie
Website: www.suicideorsurvive.ie

SpunOut.ie
SpunOut.ie is an independent, youth-powered national charity
working to empower young people to create personal and
social change.
Tel. 01 675 3554
Email: info@spunout.ie
Website: www.spunout.ie

United Kingdom

Anxiety UK
Anxiety UK works to relieve and support those living with
anxiety disorders by providing information, support and
understanding and 1:1 therapy
Zion Community Resource Centre,
339 Stretford Road, Hulme,
Manchester, M15 4ZY

Tel: 08444 775 774
Email: info@anxietyuk.org.uk
Website: www.anxietyuk.org.uk

CALM

Offers support to men in the UK, of any age, who are down or in crisis via its helpline and website.
PO Box 68766,
London, SE1P 4JZ
Tel: 0800 58 58 58
Email:info@thecalmzone.net
Website: www.thecalmzone.net

Depression Alliance

Depression Alliance is a charity in the UK for anyone affected by depression; it offers a self-help group. Depression Alliance has almost 40 years' experience in working closely with healthcare professionals and government agencies, to improve local services and to ensure a healthier, happier life for people affected by depression.
20 Great Dover Street,
London, SE1 4LX
Tel: 0845 123 23 20
Email: info@depressionalliance.org
Website: www.depressionalliance.org

Get Connected

Get Connected is a UK, free, confidential helpline for young people under 25 years of age who need help and don't know where to turn. This service is available 365 days a year.
PO Box 7777,
London, W1A 5PD
Tel: 020 7009 2500
Email: admin@getconnected.org.uk
Website: www.getconnected.org.uk

Journeys

Journeys is a support organisation based in Wales that offers support and understanding to people affected by depression, their friends, families and carers. Journeys ensures a holistic approach to overcoming depression through guided self-help, building the foundations for sustainable and long-term wellbeing. It provides information, practical resources, services and training that promote the development of skills and strategies to help people find their own route to recovery.
38 Albany Road,
Cardiff, CF24 3RQ
Tel: 029 2069 2891
Email: info@journeysonline.org.uk
Website: www.journeysonline.org.uk

Mind

Mind provides advice and support to empower anyone experiencing a mental health problem. It also campaigns to improve services, raise awareness and promote understanding.
15-19 Broadway, Stratford,
London, E15 4BQ
Tel: 020 8519 2122
Email: contact@mind.org.uk
Website: www.mind.org.uk

National Self-Harm Network

This UK charity offers individuals who self-harm support and also provides support and to family and carers of individuals who self-harm.
PO Box 7264,
Nottingham, NG1 6WJ
Tel: 0800 622 6000
Email: info@nshn.co.uk
Website: www.nshn.co.uk

PAPYRUS

Papyrus provides confidential support and advice to young people and anyone worried about a young person. They run a national helpline, HOPELineUK, including text and email services, staffed by a team of mental health professionals who provide practical help and advice to vulnerable young people and to those concerned about any young person who may be at risk of suicide.

67 Bewsey Street, Warrington,
Cheshire, WA2 7JQ
Tel: 01925 572 444
Email: admin@papyrus-uk.org
Website: www.papyrus-uk.org

Petal Support

Petal Support provides practical and emotional support, advocacy, group support and counselling for the families and friends of those who died by suicide.

8 Barrack Street,
Hamilton, ML3 0DG
Tel: 01698 324502
Email: info@petalsupport.com
Website: www.petalsupport.com

Rethink

Rethink is one of largest voluntary sector providers of mental health services with over 200 services in England. Founded 40 years ago through voluntary groups for people affected by mental illness, they have over 100 groups in England.

Rethink Mental Illness,
89 Albert Embankment,
London, SE1 7TP
Tel: 0300 5000 927
Email: advice@rethink.org
Website: www.rethink.org

Appendix

Samaritans UK

Samaritans is a confidential emotional support service for anyone in the UK and Ireland. The service is available 24 hours a day for people who are experiencing feelings of distress or despair, including those which may lead to suicide. Details below are for the central office but visit the website to find your local branch.

Freepost RSRB-KKBY-CYJK, Chris,
PO Box 90 90, Stirling, FK8 2SA
Tel (central): 08457 90 90 90
Email: jo@samaritans.org
Website: www.samaritans.org

Selfharm.co.uk

Selfharm is a charity that has developed a strong and professional reputation for delivering caring, child-centred work which focuses on the emotional and social needs of all young people.

Selfharm,
3a Upper George Street, Luton,
Bedfordshire, LU1 2QX
Email: info@selfharm.co.uk
Website: www.selfharm.co.uk

Support Line UK

Support Line UK offers confidential emotional support to children, young adults and adults by telephone, email and post. It assists people to develop healthy, positive coping strategies, an inner feeling of strength and increased self-esteem to encourage healing, recovery and moving forward with life. It also provides details of counsellors, agencies and support groups throughout the UK.

PO Box 2860, Romford,
Essex, RM7 1JA

Tel: 01708 765200
Email: info@supportline.org.uk
Website: www.supportline.org.uk

Survivors of Bereavement by Suicide

Survivors of Bereavement by Suicide is a self-help organisation that provides a confidential environment in which bereaved people can share their experiences and feelings, so giving and gaining support from each other.
Flamsteed Centre,
Albert Street, Ilkeston,
Derbyshire, DE7 5GU
Tel: 0115 944 1117
Email: sobs.admin@care4free.net
Website: www.uk-sobs.org.uk

YoungMinds

YoungMinds is the UK's leading charity committed to improving the emotional wellbeing and mental health of children and young people. Driven by their experiences, they campaign, research and influence policy and practice.
Suite 11, Baden Place, Crosby Row,
London, SE1 1YW
Tel: 020 7089 5050
Email: ymenquiries@youngminds.org.uk
Website: www.youngminds.org.uk

Youth Access

Youth Access is the national membership organisation for young people's information, advice, counselling and support services. It provides a holistic response to young people's social, emotional and mental health needs through a range of services, including social welfare advice, advocacy, counselling, health clinics, community education and personal support.

1-2 Taylors Yard, 67 Alderbrook Road,
London, SW12 8AD
Tel: 020 8772 9900
Email: admin@youthaccess.org.uk
Website: www.youthaccesa.org.uk

Specific to Scotland

Breathing Space
Breathing Space is a free, confidential phone and web-based
service for people in Scotland experiencing low mood,
depression or anxiety.
Tel: 0800 83 85 87
Email: info@breathingspacescotland.co.uk
Website: www.breathingspacescotland.co.uk

Hands on Scotland
This website aims to help you make a difference to children and
young people's lives. It gives practical information, tools and
activities to respond helpfully to troubling behaviour and to
help children and young people to flourish.
Email: handson@nhs.net
Website: www.handsonscotland.co.uk

Lifelink Services
Lifelink offers a range of stress services for adults and young
people in communities and schools across Glasgow City.
Unit E3, 145 Charles Street,
Royston, G21 2QA
Tel: 0141 552 4434
Email: info@lifelink.co.uk
Website: www.lifelink.co.uk

References and Bibliography

Amminger PG, Schafer MR, Papageorgiou K, Klier CM, Cotton SM, Harrigan SM, Berger GE. (2010) Long-chain □-3 fatty acids for indicated prevention of psychotic disorders. *Archives of General Psychiatry*; **67**(2): 146-154.

Baumrind D. (1966) Effects of Authoritative Parental Control on Child Behaviour. *Child Development*; **37**(4): 887-907.

Brendstrup E, Launse L. (1997) *Headache and Reflexological Treatment*. The Council Concerning Alternative Treatment. The National Board of Health, Denmark.

Brough N, Stewart-Brown S, Thistlethwaite J, Lindenmeyer A, Lewith G. (2012) Exploring clients' experiences of craniosacral therapy: a qualitative study. *European Journal of Integrative Medicine*; **5**(6): 575.

Brown RA, Ramsey SE, Strong DR, Myers MG, Kahler CW, Lejuex CW, *et al.* (2003) Effects of motivational interviewing on smoking cessation in adolescents with psychiatric disorders. *Tobacco Control*; Dez; **12**(Suppl IV).

Cooke H, Schneider K, Verne J. (2011) *Suicide and Self-Harm in the South West*. South West Public Health Observatory: NHS South West.

Deliberate Self Harm Annual Report (2012). Cork: National Suicide Research Foundation.

Diego MA, Field T, Hernandez-Reif M, Shaw JA, Rothe EM,

Castellanos D, Mesner L. (2002) Aggressive adolescents benefit from massage therapy. *Adolescence*; **37**: 597-607.

Edge JA. (2003) Pilot study addressing the effect of aromatherapy massage on mood, anxiety and relaxation in mental health. *Complementary Therapies in Nursing and Midwifery*; **9**: 90-97.

Field T, Morrow C, Valdeon C, Larson S, Kuhn C, Schanberg S. (1992) Massage reduces anxiety in child and adolescent psychiatric patients. *Journal of the American Academy of Child and Adolescent Psychiatry*; **31**: 125-131.

Goyal M, Singh S, Sibinga EMS, Gould NF, Rowland-Seymour A *et al.* (2014) Meditation programs for psychological stress and well-being. *JAMA Internal Medicine*; **174**(3): 357-368.

Griffin E, Arensman E, Wall A, Corcoran P, Perry IJ. (2013) *National Registry of Deliberate Self Harm Annual Report 2012*. Cork: National Suicide Research Foundation.

Groves S, Backers HS, van den Bosch W, Miller A. (2012) Review: Dialectical behaviour therapy with adolescents. *Child and Adolescent Mental Health*; **17**(2): 65-75.

Hallahan B, Hibbeln JR, Davis JM, Garland MR. (2007) Omega-3 fatty acid supplementation in patients with recurrent self-harm. Single-centre double-blind randomised controlled trial. *British Journal of Psychiatry*; **190**: 118-122.

Hawton K, Bergen H, Waters K, Ness J, Cooper J, Steeg S and Kapur N. (2012) Epidemiology and nature of self-harm in children and adolescents: findings from the multicentre study of self-harm in England. *European Child and Adolescent Psychiatry*, **7**, 369-377.

Kaslow N, Thompson M. (1998) Applying the criteria for empirically supported treatments to studies of psychosocial interventions for child and adolescent depression. *Journal of Clinical Child Psychology*; **27**: 146-155.

Kazdin A, Weisz J. (1998) Identifying and developing empirically supported child and adolescent treatments. *Journal of Consulting and Clinical Psychology*; **66**: 19-36.

Kim JS, Franklin C. (2009) Solution-focused brief therapy in schools: A review of the outcome literature. *Children and Youth Services Review*; **31**(4): 464-470.

Kübler-Ross E. (1969) *On Death and Dying*. New York: Macmillan.

Kunz B, Kunz K. (2009) *Evidence-based reflexology for health professionals and researchers*. RRP Press (The Reflexology Research Series)

Lamborn SD, Mants NS, Steinberg L, Dornbusch SM. (1991) Patterns of competence and adjustment among adolescents from authoritative, authoritarian, indulgent, and neglectful families. *Child Development*; **62**: 1049-1065.

Lee SH, Ahn SC, Lee YJ *et al.* (2007) Effectiveness of a meditation-based stress management program as an adjunct to pharmacotherapy in patients with anxiety disorder. *Journal of Psychosomatic Research*; **62**: 189-195.

Liem, J, Cavell E, Lustig K. (2010) The influence of authoritative parenting during adolescence on depressive symptoms in young adulthood: examining the mediating roles of self-development and peer support. *Journal of Genetic Psychology*; **171**(1): 73-92.

Madge N, Hewitt A, Hawton K, de Wilde E, Corcoran P, Fekete S, van Heeringen K, De Leo D, Ystgaard M. (2008) Deliberate self-harm within an international community sample of young people: comparative findings from the Child and Adolescent Self-harm in Europe (CASE) Study. *Journal of Child Psychology and Psychiatry*; **49**(6): 667-677.

Mukaino Y, Park J, White A, Ernst E. (2005) The effectiveness of acupuncture for depression. A systematic review of randomised controlled trials. *Acupuncture in Medicine*; **23**(2): 70-6.

Murphy T. (2001) *The Angry Child: Regaining Control When Your Child Is Out of Control*. Three Rivers Press: New York.

National Registry of Self-harm in Northern Ireland West (2010)

Northern Ireland Registry of Deliberate Self-Harm, Western Area: Annual Report 2009. Belfast: Department of Health Social Services and Public Safety in Northern Ireland.

Neece CL, Berk MS, Combs-Ronto LA. (2013) Dialectical behaviour therapy and suicidal behavior in adolescence: linking developmental theory and practice. *Professional Psychology: Research and Practice*; **44**(4): 257-265.

Payne S, Horn S, Relf M. (2010) *Loss and Bereavement*. UK: Open University Press.

Rando TA. (1993) *Treatment of Complicated Mourning*. USA: BookCrafters

Shear K, Frank E, Houck P, Reynolds C. (2005) Treatment of complicated grief: A randomized controlled trial. *JAMA*; **293**: 2601-2608.

Smith C, Hancock H, Blake-Mortimer J, Eckert K. (2007) A randomised comparative trial of yoga and relaxation to reduce stress and anxiety. *Complementary Therapeutic Medicine*; **15**(2): 77-83. (Epub 2006 Jun 21.)

Stroebe M, Schut H. (1999) The dual process model of coping with bereavement: rationale and description. *Death Studies*; **23**: 197-224.

Testa GW. (2000) A study on the effects of reflexology on migraine headaches. http://members.tripod.com/GTesta/Dissertationall.htm. (Accessed on 24 February 2014.)

Whitlock J, Eckenrode J, Silverman D. (2006) Self-injurious behaviours in a college population. *Pediatrics*;**117**:1939-1948.

Wolfradt U, Hempel S, Miles JNV. (2003) Perceived parenting styles, depersonalisation, anxiety and coping behaviour in adolescents. *Personality and Individual Differences*; **34**(3): 521-532.

Worden WJ. (1991) *Grief counselling and grief therapy: A handbook for the mental health practitioner* (2nd edition). London: Springer.

Worden WJ. (2005) *Grief Counselling and Grief Therapy* (3rd edition). East Sussex, England: Routledge.

World Health Organization Suicide prevention (SUPRE). Available at: http://www.who.int/mental_health/prevention/suicide/suicideprevent/en/ (Accessed on 18 March 2014).

Index

A&E, discharge following
    attempted suicide, 38
abuse, 40–42
    sexual, 18, 40–41
acceptance of/adjustment to
    one's child's suicide, 121,
    122
ACCEPTS technique, 64–65
Accident & Emergency
    (A&E), discharge
    following attempted
    suicide, 38
acknowledgment of loss of
    child, 121–122
acupuncture, 85–87
adjustment to/acceptance of
    loss of child, 121, 122
Adler, Alfred, 105, 106
affirmation *see*
    encouragement
aggression and massage, 80
AID (acronym), 25, 26
alcohol misuse, 43, 45
alopecia, 18
alpha-linolenic acid (ALA),
    92–93
alternative and
    complementary therapies,
    73–91
amino acids, 93
anger

at death of one's child,
    130
    teenager, 9–10, 111–115
antidepressants, 8, 19
anxiety, 8–9, 115–118
    essential oils, 82
    fight or flight response
    and, 8, 84, 115
    massage, 80–81
    meditation, 88
    mindfulness, 88
    parenting and, 115–118
    reflexology, 78
    stress, 89
Anxiety UK, 137–138
apologies, 68
Applied Suicide Intervention
    Skills Training (ASIST),
    46–47
ARM (acronym), 25, 26
aromatherapy, 81–83
ascorbic acid (vitamin C),
    98–99
ASIST (Applied Suicide
    Intervention Skills
    Training), 46–47
assumption questions, 60
attention seeking, 27, 32
authoritarian parenting,
    109–110
authoritative parenting,

110–111
autonomic nervous system and craniosacral therapy and, 84
Aware, 133

bargaining following loss of child, 130–131
basil oil, 82
behavioural reaction to threat, 116
beliefs, negative/irrational, 58
bereavement (loss by death)
    by suicide
    parents coping with, 119–131
    support/self-help group, 142
    teenager coping with, 39–40
    suicide risk with, 33
bergamot oil, 82
biotin (vitamin B7), 97–98
bisexuality, 42
biting, 17
black and white thinking, 59
body bashing, 19–20
bonded (feeling), 105
Breathing Space, 143
bullying, 43
burning, 17

caffeine, 102–103
calcium, 100–101
CALM, 138
cannabis, 74
carbohydrate (including sugar)
    complex, 92, 103
    refined, 91, 101–102, 103
CASE (Child and Adolescent Self-harm in Europe) Study, 23
catastrophising, 58

cedar wood oil, 82
cerebrospinal fluid and craniosacral therapy, 84
change talk, 72–74
child abuse see abuse
Child and Adolescent Self-harm in Europe (CASE) Study, 23
clarifying questions, 59–60
clary sage oil, 82
cobalamin (vitamin B12), 98
cognitive behavioural therapy (CBT), 8, 57–62
competent (feeling), 105
complementary therapies, 73–91
compliments see encouragement
congruence, 51, 68
consequences and implications questions, 61
Console, 134
coping (skills/strategies)
    self-harm, 26–27
    solution-based brief therapy, 53–54
coriander oil, 82
cortisol, 89, 99
counselling and counsellors, 50–51
    bereavement, 127–128
craniosacral therapy, 83–85
CRAP foods, 66, 91
crisis management, 28
cutting, 16–17, 20

DARN-CAT process, 73–74
DEARMAN technique, 67
death see bereavement; suicide
defeatism see self-defeatist syndrome
dehydration, 94, 103
democratic parenting, 106–107
denial in death of one's child,

130
depression, 7–8
    acupuncture, 86–87,
    91–104
    anxiety and, 8–9
    bereaved parents, 121,
    129
    essential oils, 82–83
    massage, 80–81
    meditation, 88
Depression Alliance, 138
dialectical behaviour therapy,
    63–70
diet/eating/food/nutrition,
    4–5, 86–87, 91–104
    supplements, 10, 95, 96,
    97, 104
distraction, ACCEPTS
    method, 64–65
distress, 1, 10, 15, 17, 20, 28
    bereaved parent, 127
    suicide and, 32, 34, 39, 42,
    43
    therapies addressing, 63,
    65, 69
divorce and separation,
    parental, 35–36
docosahexaenoic acid (DHA),
    92–93, 94, 95, 96
drugs
    misuse, 43, 45, 67, 74
    overdose and poisoning,
    19, 21, 22
    prescribed see medication

eating see diet
eicosapentaenoic acid (EPA),
    92–93, 94, 95, 96
emotion(s), 118
    anger and, 112
    negative, managing, 64
    painful see pain
    reasoning with, 59
    regulation of, 63, 68–69

story of, 69–70
empathy, 24, 25, 34, 37, 111,
    116, 117
    bereavement, 122, 127,
    130
    therapist, 51, 52, 68, 71, 72
encouragement (incl.
    affirmation/compliments/
    validation), 37, 68
    bereaved parents, 127
    in cognitive behavioural
    therapy, 62
    in dialectical behaviour
    therapy, 64, 65, 66, 67, 68,
    70
    in motivational
    interviewing, 71, 72
    in parenting, 106, 107,
    108, 110, 117, 118
    in solution-based therapy,
    52, 53, 56–57
energy, low, 3–4
engagement with life,
    bereaved parents, 129
essential fats, 92–93, 94–96
essential oils and
    aromatherapy, 81–83
evidence and reason
    questions, 60–61
excoriation disorder, 17
exercise, 26, 67, 103

family members
    death, 33–34
        by suicide, 39–40
    sexual abuse involving,
    41
    support following
    attempted suicide, 38–39
    see also parents
FAST techniques, 68
fats and fatty acids
    essential, 92–93, 94–96
    trans, 94, 102

fight or flight response, 8, 84, 99, 115
filtering, 58
fish, 95–96, 97, 98
    oily, and fish oil, 94, 95
folic acid or folate (vitamin B9), 98
food *see* diet
frankincense, 82
free-radicals, 96, 99
friend(s)
    death, 33–34
        by suicide, 39–40
    separation from (by moving to a new location), 36
    see also peers
FRIEND-TER-VENTION, 46, 47

gamma linoleic acid, 10
gay teenagers, 42
geranium oil, 82–83
Get Connected, 138
GIVE skills, 68
'Gremlin', 1, 2, 3, 5, 105
    dealing with/evicting, 12, 65, 68, 69, 118
    depression and, 8
    self-esteem and, 6, 7
grief in suicide
    adolescent's (loss of friend or family member), 49–50
    parents', 119, 120–127
GROW, 134

hair, pulling out, 18
Hands on Scotland, 143
haplessness, 45
head banging, 19
head massage, Indian, 76–77
headache, 78–79, 84
    migraine, 83, 84, 85, 96,

100
    tension, 8, 9, 76, 77, 78–79, 80
    water and, 94, 103
Headstrong, 134
HeadsUp, 135
healing of wounds, interfering with, 30
help *see* support and help
helplessness
    bereaved parents, 126, 127, 129, 130
    teenager, 44, 45, 54, 59
heterosexuality, 42
hitting, 18, 30
holistic and complementary therapies, 73–91
home move to new location, 36–37
homework in CBT, 62
homosexuality, 42
HOPE intervention, 46, 47
hopelessness
    bereaved parents, 127, 130
    teenager, 1, 7, 33, 44, 45, 126
hormones and acupuncture, 86
hospital discharge following attempted suicide, 38
house move to new location, 36–37

imagery in dialectical behaviour therapy, 65
implications and consequences questions, 61
IMPROVE (acronym), 65–66
Indian head massage, 76–77
interpersonal effectiveness, 63
Ireland
    help and support, 133–137

National Registry of
Deliberate Self-Harm, 21
isolation (social)
parents of suicide victim,
128–129
suicide risk and, 33, 34,
37, 39, 40, 43, 45

Journeys, 139

Kübler-Ross's five stages of
grief, 120–121

labelling, negative, 114
lavender oil, 83
lemongrass oil, 83
lesbian teenagers, 42
life and living (following loss
of child), 121, 122, 123, 124,
125, 127, 128, 129, 130, 131
Lifelink Services, 143
lifestyle, 4–5
□-linoleic acid, 10
□-linolenic acid (ALA), 92–93
loss
by death *see* bereavement
suicide due to, 33–38

magnesium, 100
massage, 79–81
aromatherapy, 81
Indian head, 76–77
mastery, 67
meaning in dialectical
behaviour therapy, 65
medical disorder/physical
illness, 3–4, 66, 77
medication (prescribed drugs)
depression, 8
monitoring/supervision/
taking control of, 19, 39
meditation, 87–88
mindful (mindfulness),
63, 87, 88

Mental Health Ireland, 135
mental illness (mental health
problems; psychological/
psychiatric disorder), 26,
31–32, 32
foods and, 101–102
massage, 80–81
sources of help, 134–135,
136, 137, 139, 140, 142
micronutrients
minerals, 93–94, 100–101
vitamins, 93–94, 96–100
migraine, 83, 84, 85, 96, 100
Mind, 139
mind-reading, 59
mindfulness (mindful
meditation), 63, 87, 88
minerals, 93–94, 100–101
miracle questions, 55–56
mood and food, 92–101,
102–103
motivational interviewing,
70–74
mourning by parents after
suicide, 120, 121–123
moving to a new location,
36–37

National Registry of
Deliberate Self-Harm
Ireland, 21
National Registry of
Deliberate Self-Harm
Northern Ireland West, 22
National Self-Harm Network,
139
negative emotions, managing,
64
negative labelling, 114
negative thoughts/thinking/
cognitions, 115
combating/challenging/
managing, 57–62, 65, 69,
86, 117

depression, 7
sleeplessness and, 5
triggers/activating
events, 58
nervous system
acupuncture, 86
autonomic, craniosacral
therapy and, 84
niacin (vitamin B3), 97
Northern Ireland, National
Registry of Deliberate Self-
Harm in Western area, 22
nutrition *see* diet

OARS technique, 72
omega-3 fatty acids, 92, 93,
94–95, 102
omega-6 fatty acids, 92, 93
origin and sources questions,
61
osteopathy, cranial, 83–85
over-generalising, 58
over-rubbing of skin, 19
overwhelming feelings
bereaved parents, 127,
129
teenagers, 18, 35, 54, 113,
118

pain (emotional)
bereaved parents, 121,
122, 125, 127, 130, 131
suicide due to, 33, 34, 35,
37
pantothenic acid (vitamin B5),
97
Papyrus, 140
paracetamol overdose, 22
parent(s)
bereavement through
suicide, 119–131
separation, 35–36
taking on discovery of
self-harming, 25, 35–36

see also family members
parenting, 105–118
styles, 106–111
peers
rejection by, 37–38
relationships, 34
see also friends
peppermint oil, 83
permissive parenting, 107–109
personalising, 58
perspective and viewpoint
questions, 61–62
Petal Support, 140
phone coaching, 64
physical abuse, 40
physical activity/exercise, 26,
67, 103
physical illness/medical
disorder, 3–4, 66, 77
physiological reaction to
threat, 115–116
picking skin, 17
Pieta House, 135–136
pinching, 18, 20
PLEASE MASTER (acronym),
66–67
poisoning (incl. drugs
overdose), 19, 21, 22
polarised thinking, 59
poly-unsaturates, 92
positive regard, unconditional,
51
positive reinforcement, *see also*
encouragement
potassium, 101
prayer in dialectical behaviour
therapy, 65
pre-menstrual tension, 10, 82,
93, 97
prescribed drugs, 39
problem-solving, 113
competency, 62
instant, 114
self-help technique, 28

professionals
   discovery of self-
   harming, 25
   self-harm interventions
   skill training, 27–28
   talk therapy, 49–50
protein, 93
psychiatrist, 50
psychological disorder/
   psychiatric illness *see*
   mental illness
psychological reaction to
   threat, 115
psychological treatment (talk
   therapies), 5, 8, 29, 49–74
psychologist, 50
psychotherapist, 50
punching, 18
pyridoxine (vitamin B6), 97

Qi, 85
questions (therapists')
   cognitive behavioural
   therapy, 59–62
   motivational
   interviewing, 72, 73
   solution-based brief
   therapy, 53–56

Reach Out, 136
reason and evidence
   questions, 60–61
reflections, 53, 72
reflexology, 77–79
relationship (romantic), break
   up, 34–35
relaxation in dialectical
   behaviour therapy, 65
ReThink, 140
riboflavin (vitamin B2), 96
risk assessment, self-harm, 28
risk factors
   self-defeatist syndrome,
   11–12

suicide, 33–43
romantic relationship, break
   up, 34–35
rosemary oil, 83
rules and parenting, 106, 107,
   108, 109, 115

Samaritans, UK and Ireland,
   136, 141
scaling questions, 55
school, 44
   bullying, 43
   moving to new one, 36,
   37
   solution-based brief
   therapy, 52
Scotland, help and support,
   143
scratching, 17, 20
self, sense of, 1–2
self-defeatist syndrome
   consequences, 13–29,
   31–47
   parenting, 105–118
   understanding, 1–12
self-esteem, low, 6–7
self-harm, 10–11, 13–29
   acts/methods, 15–21
   complications, 21
   coping strategies, 26–27
   interventions skill
   training, 27–28
   prevalence, 21–22
   reasons behind act of,
   14–15
   signs, 23–24
   taking action on
   discovery, 24–25
   understanding, 13–14
Selfharm.co.uk, 141
self-will, 2
sensations in dialectical
   behaviour therapy, 65
separation

from friends (by moving
to a new location), 36
parental, 35–36
serotonin, 101-102
sexual abuse, 18, 40–41
sexual orientation, 42–43
Shine, 136–137
signs and symptoms
bereaved parents'
complicated grief,
126–127
self-defeatist syndrome, 3
self-harm, 23–24
suicidal thoughts, 44–45
sleep, 5, 67
social isolation *see* isolation
social networking sites, 39–40
Socratic questioning, 59–62
solution-based brief therapy,
52–57
SOS - Suicide or Survive, 137
sources and origin questions,
61
SpunOut.ie, 137
starflower oil, 10
STOP intervention, 46, 47
Storm (Self-Harm Intervention
Skills Training), 27–28
stress, 1, 99
complementary therapies
relieving, 75, 76, 77, 78,
84, 84–85, 86, 87, 88, 89
exercise and sunlight
and, 103
minerals and, 101
vitamins and, 96, 97, 99
substance (drug) misuse, 43,
45, 67, 74
sugar, blood, 92, 97, 99, 101,
103
see also carbohydrate
suicide, 31–47, 119–131
bereavement by *see*
bereavement

of friend or family
member, 39–40
myths, 32–33
prior attempts, 38–39
risk factors, 33–43
thinking of (ideation), 9,
11, 31, 32, 34, 35, 40, 42,
44–45, 74
Suicide or Survive (SOS), 137
S.U.I.C.I.D.E (acronym),
128–129
summarising in motivational
interviewing, 72
sunlight, 103
supplements (dietary), 10, 95,
96, 97, 104
support and help, 133–137
anxious teenagers,
116–118
attempted suicide, 38–39
bereaved parents,
129–131
moving to new location,
37
professional *see*
professionals
sources, 133–137
Support Line UK, 141–142
Survivors of Bereavement by
Suicide, 142
symptoms *see* signs and
symptoms
syndrome, meaning, 3

talk therapies, 5, 8, 29, 49–74
key models, 52–74
main tenets, 51
talking about suicide, 32
therapies, talk, 5, 8, 29, 49–74
thiamine (vitamin B1), 96
thoughts/thinking
negative *see* negative
thoughts/thinking
suicidal, 9, 11, 31, 32, 34,

35, 40, 42, 44–45, 74
3Ts, 133
trans fats, 94, 102
trichotillomania, 18

unconditional positive regard,
    51
United Kingdom, help and
    support, 137–143

vacation in dialectical
    behaviour therapy, 65
validation *see* encouragement
values, core, 2, 68, 71
viewpoint and perspective
    questions, 61–62
vitamins, 93–94, 96–100

water, 94, 103
    dehydration, 94, 103
WHO *see* World Health
    Organisation
Worden's four tasks of
    mourning, 121–122
World Health Organisation
    (WHO)
        definition of self-harm, 14
        suicide statistics, 31
wound healing, interfering
    with, 30

ylang ylang oil, 83
yoga, 89–90
YoungMinds, 142
Youth Access, 142–143

zinc, 101

About the Author

Liz Quish is a qualified and highly experienced counsellor, psychotherapist, parent coach, early childhood educator and mediator. She has been working with children and families for over 20 years, more recently as a Crisis Counsellor, supporting and counselling teenagers and adults who present with self-harm and suicidal thinking.

Liz has a wealth of knowledge and skills in relation to appropriate interventions and support for those in suicidal distress and who engage in self-harming, with very positive outcomes. She is also a highly regarded lecturer and facilitates workshops and trainingprogrammes in the following areas:

- Understanding and Managing Anger in a proactive manner
- Stress Management
- Mindfulness for Wellness
- Child Development
- Child Protection
- Positive and Productive Parenting
- Self Esteem
- Conflict Coaching
- Staff Supervision and Development in Early Childhood Settings
- Parent Coaching
- Special Needs

Liz is available to deliver and design bespoke workshops based on specified requirements.

She can be contacted by email on liz@csei.ie

Website: www.csei.ie

Facebook: Centre for Social and Emotional Intelligence